HERE'S POWER FOR YOU

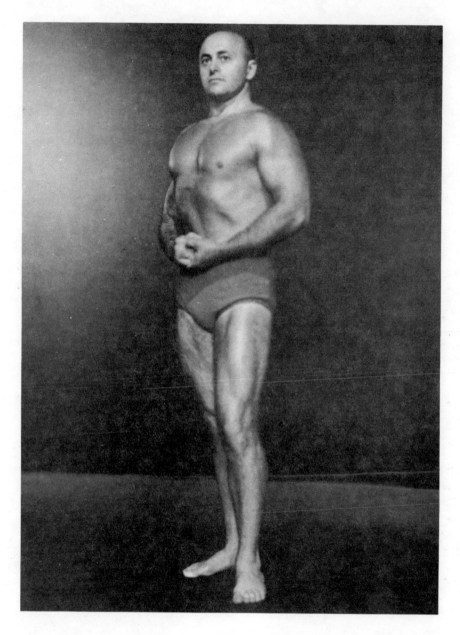

Fig. 1   Photo by Jack Sidney, Brooklyn, New York

David Manners, the author, owns and operates the Manners Health Studio in Elmont, New York. A considerable part of his time is devoted to privately teaching children corrective exercises, body building and the art of self-defense. He was formerly an artists' model for sculpture and painting at the School of Fine Arts at Yale University.

HERE'S POWER FOR YOU

Complete body-building courses. Special instruction for boys and adults—for the overweight and underweight. Calisthenics. How to exercise with Bar-bells, Dumb-bells, and Pulleys.

David Manners

ARCO PUBLISHING, INC.
NEW YORK

Acknowledgments:

The author is grateful to Sylvia Manners, his wife, for her devoted assistance preparing the manuscript.

Photographs of athletes appearing on pages 34, 51, 58, 62, 63, 68, 73, 92, 98, 100, 105, 112 and 117—courtesy of *Body Builder Magazine*. Exercise photographs by Jack Sidney, Brooklyn, New York and Charles Berman, West Hempstead, New York.

Revised Edition

Seventh Arco Printing, 1981

Published by Arco Publishing , Inc.
219 Park Avenue South, New York, N.Y. 10003

Library of Congress Catalog Card Number 74-29790
ISBN 0-668-03242-1

Printed in the United States of America

CONTENTS

INTRODUCTION

ANYBODY CAN develop muscles and build up his body. Many people have the mistaken idea that physical strength and a well-formed body can only be inherited. This is not the whole truth. While some of us may inherit a well-formed physique, the frail and weak need not remain underdeveloped. By following a well-planned progressive course of exercises the average person can, within three months, increase his chest measurement by 2 inches, arms by one inch, neck by one inch, thighs by 2 inches, and calves by one inch. His weight can increase from 5 to 20 pounds. He can double his strength within 6 months.

In my first 18 months of training, I gained *40 pounds*, from 125 to 165. This experience is not out of the ordinary.

Psychiatrists are becoming increasingly aware of the importance of a well-formed body for emotional stability, and they frequently prescribe body building exercise for boys and young men, to help reduce timidity, self-consciousness and fear.

Fully matured men, well past their athletic prime, tend to forget that their bodies require regular exercise to remain in good condition. A few years after they have ceased to train, their physical condition begins to deteriorate. Poor diet, drinking, smoking, late hours and not enough rest contribute to this process. As we enter middle age, we fall prey to many ailments that could have been avoided, had we paid more attention to our physical condition.

We know that exercise is good for us. Most of us have, at one time or another, experienced the exhilaration, the feeling of being alive, healthy, and full of pep, that comes from possessing a well-conditioned body.

Our intentions are always good. We appreciate the need for keeping fit; yet somehow, we just can't get started. The daily routine of getting up in the morning, going to work, coming

7

home, eating dinner, reading an evening newspaper, and watching television before going off to sleep, tends to weaken our good intentions.

None the less, we cannot afford to let ourselves drift into a weakened, sluggish and overweight condition. Common excuses like "no time," or "too tired," or, "I don't want to begin an exercise I will have to continue for the rest of my life" are poor excuses indeed. The 2 or 3 hours a week that you allot for physical improvement and conditioning is the best and the most inexpensive investment you can make. It pays large dividends in health, strength, a well-formed body, and physical well-being. Your body is like a machine. It will deteriorate and break down if not given proper attention. You can't trade it for a later model, like a car. Make up your mind to adopt an exercise routine and do it consistently. You will be amazed at the results.

Exercise need not be looked upon as a chore, as something that must be gotten over with. There are millions of enthusiastic people all over the world who have successfully made physical culture their hobby. Why not make it yours?

The way in which exercise affects the human body is in itself a remarkable phenomenon. If you are a beginner, you will marvel at the transformation of your average or underdeveloped body into a well-formed physique, with improved bodily carriage and posture. A strong, healthy body gives you confidence to face the ordeals and conflicts of daily living. Many other people, who are afraid of sickness and the infirmities of old age, will find the secret to the fountain of youth in regular exercise, proper diet and rest. It will definitely keep you from growing old.

Most movie actors maintain their youthful and attractive appearance by exercising regularly. If they did not take care of themselves, the public would soon lose interest in them.

The condition of your body is the barometer of the appearance of your face. It will retain its youthful appearance for a longer period, if your body is healthy and well-conditioned.

Remember that our bodies are always in a state of change. Either we improve, or we deteriorate. Make up your mind to improve. Begin your training, and stick to it. In a few months, you will be more than satisfied with the results.

Chapter 1

How to exercise with weights

IT IS only natural for the enthusiastic beginner to overdo it. The following morning he wakes up with muscular aches and pains, and vows never to exercise again. These aches and pains can be avoided if you follow the courses of exercises as outlined in the book. You will experience only a minimum of muscular soreness.

The proper method for training with weights is to exercise 3 times a week, every other day. You might exercise Monday, Wednesday and Friday, or Tuesday, Thursday and Saturday, or, whatever alternate days you choose. When you exercise your muscles, you break down your tissues. You need a rest day to give your tissues a chance to rebuild. That is why you should exercise on alternate days.

The best time to exercise is at three or four o'clock in the afternoon, or in the evening, an hour or two after dinner. If, however, the afternoons or evenings are not suitable, exercise whenever it is convenient. It is not advisable to exercise immediately after eating. You should give your food a chance to be digested. Wait an hour or two before your workout. After your workout, wait at least a half hour to an hour before you eat. When you exercise, the heart pumps blood to those muscles that are being used, and the blood requires this time to normalize before it is used to help proper digestion.

Before beginning the courses of exercises, check your weight and have someone take your measurements. Note these measurements on page 126. If possible, take a snapshot of yourself and mount it on page 128. Recheck your weight and measurements each month. In this way, you will know exactly what improvement you are making. Whether you train in a gym or in your own home, try to exercise before a mirror. Thus, you can see whether you are doing the exercises properly, and also watch the improvement of your physique.

To avoid muscle strain, the exercise room must be properly ventilated and comfortably warm. The temperature should be at least 65 to 70 degrees. When you are working out, wear a sweat shirt or any clothing that will keep you warm. There are very few athletes who do not keep warm before they participate in sports. Warm muscles respond quickly to exercise, and there is less likelihood of straining your muscles.

Before beginning any exercise, warm up by pressing the bar, without weights, a few times, and then do some deep knee-bends with the bar. If you have never lifted any weights before, begin with a light weight, 30 or 40 pounds. If you can press this weight overhead 8 or 10 times comfortably, then it is the proper weight for you. Let us say that you have decided to start with 40 pounds. Use this weight for the entire week. Perform 8 to 10 repetitions for a given exercise. The following week, add one or 2 repetitions to your exercises as indicated in the instructions. When you can repeat the exercise 12 to 15 times, you are ready to increase the weight by 3 to 5 pounds, according to your strength. You will find that for certain exercises, such as the deep knee-bend and the dead lift, which involve the thighs, hips and back, you can increase the weight by 10 to 15 pounds, because the muscles involved are the largest and strongest in the body.

Do each exercise correctly. There is a tendency among body builders to use more weight than they can properly manage. You derive more benefit if you do your exercises correctly with a lighter weight, than incorrectly with a heavier weight.

After your workout take a warm shower. This is very conducive to sleep. If you plan to go outdoors, take a warm shower and gradually turn it cool, so that there will be less chance of catching cold.

A beginner's workout should not take longer than a half hour. As your body becomes accustomed to the workouts, you can gradually increase the time to an hour. By training three times a week, you should be able to develop an outstanding physique. Do not exercise to a point where you feel completely exhausted. This is detrimental to your health and will not help to build muscles. The properly completed workout will leave you comfortably tired and your muscles will feel as though they have been thoroughly exercised.

How to exercise with weights

You may have read, in weight lifting magazines, that certain outstanding body builders use tremendous weights in their training routines, like 300 to 400 pounds in the squat and in the bench press. This may be highly commendable, but it is not necessary to handle such heavy weights to develop a good physique. You can, by a gradual process, work up to moderately heavy weights, of 150 to 200 pounds in the deep knee-bend and the bench press, and to 200 to 250 pounds in the dead lift.

To those who are interested in entering physique contests, and who have the physical structure to become champions or near champions, or, to those who want to break existing weight lifting records, I say, "Go ahead. I'll enjoy reading about it." This book, however, is written for the boy or the man of average, and under average physique, who is interested in a moderate weight training program to develop a healthy, well-proportioned physique.

Training versus straining

Some people may be afraid of barbells because of the danger of possible strain and injury. If you follow the instructions in this book, there is no reason for strain or injury. Dangers exist only when the novice receives his barbell set and immediately attempts to test his strength to the limit, instead of following a carefully worked out course.

In the beginning, take enough rest between exercises. Some persons may require more rest than others. You will find that light exercises require anywhere from 30 seconds to one minute's rest. The heavy exercises may require more. We all differ in physique and stamina, and the degree of rest will depend on the individual. You may find that you need more rest between exercises when working out during the summer. It may also be wiser to cut down on exercises in hot and humid weather.

Most people, working out with barbells, seem to prefer 10 repetitions. Whether it be 10, 15, or 20, it is not absolutely essential to your development, that you complete the exact number of repetitions you set as your goal. If your goal is 10 repetitions and you feel that you cannot get beyond the 8th or 9th, don't strain and struggle for your 10th repetition. By working out regularly, the 10th repetition will come as easily as the 9th.

In this way, you will finish the workout feeling exhilarated instead of exhausted. Let me repeat, *it is not advisable to work out to the point of exhaustion.* Moderation is the answer to a safe and sensible workout.

Exercise apparatus on the market

The average person cannot be expected to know all about body building exercise apparatus. He is continuously overwhelmed with ads for stationary bicycles, rowing machines, rubber expanders and spring expanders.

You can develop your legs by the use of the stationary bicycle, if the tension of the bicycle can be progressively increased. The rowing machines will help to develop the back muscles and arms, if there is enough resistance. The expanders, both rubber and spring, are good to develop the upper body. But sooner or later the tension in these expanders will grow less, and you can never be sure whether you have become stronger, or, whether your expanders have become weaker.

A barbell set has the advantage over all of these exercises. It will develop your entire body, and you can always depend on the weight remaining the same. The price of a barbell set is modest. It will last a lifetime and always has a resale value.

Chapter 2

Underweight and overweight.
Exercise for children

THE BEGINNER who is underweight, should follow these rules:

Exercise 3 times a week on alternate days. You must exercise regularly and not miss any workouts, unless you are too tired or feel exhausted.

You must get 8 to 10 hours sleep, and you must rest as much as possible. Remain inactive; do not take part in any other strenuous activities until you have gained sufficient weight, and have developed a good physique. Then, and only then, should you resume your normal physical activities.

Your diet is an important part of your program to gain weight. You do not have to stuff yourself at each meal. You might, however, try to eat between meals. Eat an early breakfast, and then, a late breakfast, an early lunch, and then, a late lunch. If you have your dinner at 6 p.m. have a sandwich and two glasses of milk about 8 or 9 p.m. Try to cultivate the habit of drinking milk with all your meals; it is very good for weight gaining. Many of my students have gained weight by drinking 2 or more quarts of milk a day. You can also try this weight-gaining formula which is mixed in a blender: 2 glasses of milk, 1 cup of powdered milk, 2 scoops of ice cream, 1 egg and malt—a very tasty drink and most of my students like it.

Read the next paragraph carefully because it will indicate precisely those exercises that will help you gain weight. Concentrate on developing the largest muscles of the body: the thighs, hips and latissimus dorsi (see page 34). Therein lies the secret of increasing weight. These muscles will be developed by the following exercises. The squats (or knee-bends) and the leg-press develop the thighs and hips. Chinning, rowing motion with barbells (page 121), and pulleys (page 86) will develop the latissimus dorsi muscles.

Here's power for you

Progressive weight training is the only practical solution for the underweight who want to gain weight and develop a strong, muscular physique. If you try to gain weight through diet alone, you will only put on fat.

People who are overweight have a simple problem if they have the will power to follow a sensible diet. Your doctor will prescribe a proper calorie diet to help you lose weight without endangering your health. It is absolutely necessary that you obtain all the necessary food value while you are on your diet. The only scientific diet is a balanced calorie diet, whereby you know exactly how many calories you consume in one day. Your doctor will inform you exactly how many calories you may have. Since we all vary in size, health and strength, he will be the best judge of how many calories you need. The average person consumes 3000 to 4000 calories a day. By cutting down on your calorie intake you lose weight.

Most people are under the impression that they can lose weight by exercise. They play golf, handball, tennis, etc. They weigh themselves before and after their workout and find that they do lose from one to five pounds, depending on the type of workout. This loss of weight, however, is mainly water weight. It will soon be replaced by drinking liquids. The only true loss of weight is that which results from dieting. Although there is very little weight lost through exercise, it is necessary that you exercise because it improves blood circulation, it aids the digestive organs, and it is helpful to elimination. Exercise also increases your strength while dieting.

When you have succeeded in taking off the required weight, your body will look trim and muscular, instead of flabby and weak.

No one can do this for you. It is something that has to be done by you alone. Your main problem will be to stick to your diet. After you have come down to the desired weight, you might indulge yourself a little on week-ends, and resume dieting on weekdays. Moderation in eating habits is important to maintain a trim, healthy figure.

In addition to not looking well, overweight is an unhealthy condition that may shorten your life. Fat men are more susceptible to diabetes, heart trouble, high blood pressure, etc. This is good enough reason for you to diet and exercise.

Exercise for children

The question is often asked, "What is the right age to start a boy on exercise?" You can exercise your child right from the cradle. The doctor will prescribe certain exercises for the baby in various stages of growing up. As soon as the baby starts to crawl and walk, grownups do not have the energy to keep up with him. Some mothers take their child, as young as three years old, to dancing school, where they are taught acrobatics, tap and ballet. They think nothing of having their youngsters take swimming lessons. These are all vigorous exercises. Thus, without conscious planning you are giving your child physical training at a very early age.

In this book, we are primarily interested in the best age for starting your boy on progressive weight training. You may hear of some youngsters exercising from the age of four. As a rule, they are trained by fathers who have had a great deal of experience in this field. The best time to start your son is about ten years of age. At this period he becomes aware of his physical make-up. Through physical contact with friends and foe, he appreciates the value of a strong, well-developed body. Parents are beginning to understand the importance of building the self-confidence of their boy through a program of exercise that strengthens his body. Enroll your son for a course at a competent barbell gym, where he will receive proper instructions. If this is not possible, then you, as parents, can do a great deal to help him. When your son first receives his barbell set he should be watched carefully. No doubt he will try to lift more than is good for him. He must be made to understand that the weights, when properly used, will be of great benefit to him. It is up to the parent to read the instructions in this book, and guide his son until he understands exactly how to follow the course on his own.

Start the boy with the empty bar (no weights attached) and gradually increase the weight by one and a quarter, or two and a half pounds (see chapter on Barbells). If your boy is underweight, he should follow a weight-gaining diet. Curtail his athletic activities until he has gained enough weight through weight training. Rest is important. He should receive from nine to ten hours sleep a day.

If your boy is overweight, he can continue with his athletic activities *together* with his weight training. His big problem is to maintain a reducing diet and to exercise regularly. By carefully observng the "big three"—*exercise, diet* and *proper rest,* your boy will be on the right road to self-confidence through strength, health and a well-developed physique.

A few words of caution:

A boy might find it tiring to complete the number of repetitions specified in the text for a given exercise. If this should be the case, it would be better for him to perform fewer repetitions in the beginning, and gradually work up to the required number over a period of a few weeks. At no time must he be permitted to strain himself. He must do the repetitions easily, and without strain. If one particular exercise becomes difficult to perform, change to another exercise requiring the use of different muscles. If the boy shows any sign of fatigue, discontinue the exercises, and let him rest a day.

Sometimes, the boy might have been playing at some sport outdoors, before he begins to exercise with weights. He may show signs of fatigue half way through the workout, although he might not be aware of it. The wise parent will stop the exercises and let him rest a day.

Most important for body development is to do the exercises correctly. Straining will definitely not build him up. Proper exercising will.

Chapter 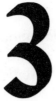 3

The ideal physique
Weight-training for sports
How Calisthenics help you

THERE ARE three general types of physical specimens that this book deals with. There is the thin, light-boned type, who find it more difficult to develop their bodies. When they finally achieve proper development, their muscular definition is the envy of those with heavier type of physiques.

Then, there is the medium type. They have the most favorable type of body to begin with, because their physiques seem to respond more readily to exercise than other types. Finally, there is the heavy-boned. They will find little trouble molding their bodies to proper proportion if they follow a sensible diet and exercise regularly.

We cannot escape our type. We are bound to our physical structure. If you are slim, don't expect to develop a massive type of physique. By exercising regularly and getting a proper amount of sleep, and adhering to a well-balanced diet, you will improve your strength and physical structure along the lines nature gave you. The same can be said of the heavy type. Don't expect to slim down to aesthetic lines. There is, however, no reason why you cannot realize your goal for a muscular body and a trim waistline.

You will find in this book photos of outstanding athletes. Choose one that most nearly resembles your type of physique. While no two bodies are exactly alike, there are similar types. Try to pattern your physique after what you consider your type. It is always best to work towards a goal. Visualize what you want to look like, and work for it.

The most essential thing we must all strive for is a physique that is in proper proportion. There is a tendency for the underweight body builder to overdo it, when he finally gains weight and develops a good physique. There appears to be a drive in the body building field to develop mountains of muscle, regardless of the individual's height and proportion. Certain measurements are held up to us as the supreme goal, like a 19 inch arm, a 50 inch chest or 27 inch thighs. There are some physical specimens in the body building field who have these measurements. Some have the height, and the mass of muscle looks well on them. Others, however, look as though they were foreshortened and out of proportion. Developing an arm that looks like a side of beef, and developing thighs that are so huge that they swerve from side to side when you walk, is hardly the answer to a well-developed physique.

What do you strive for in developing an ideal physique? The proportion of your body should be *well-balanced*. The lower half of your body should be in proportion to the upper half of your body. Your muscles need not measure to a magic number like 16 or 18 inch arms, or 26 to 28 inch thighs. The tape does not tell the entire story, but your eyes do, and the eyes of other people do. The quality and appearance of a muscle is more important than tape measurement.

Abdominals and external obliques (see page 34) must receive special attention. No matter how well your body may be developed, unless these muscles are well-defined and free from fat, your physique will lose a great deal in appearance. If you keep your waistline trim, you will always be in good shape.

Weight training for sports

This section is prepared expressly for the reader who is interested in weight training as a means of improving his performance in other sports. Training with weights has been proven to be the quickest and best method to build up your body. Since most of our training is done in a stationary position, there is hardly any real movement, like running forward and backward, or running from side to side as in handball or tennis. All of the physical activity is confined to a small floor space, 6 feet by 6 feet. While you can achieve agility and coordination through weight lifting, you will obtain far better results by combining weight lifting with the sport you are interested in, like tennis and handball.

In the beginning, the underweight should refrain from participating in any sport. Wait until you have gained enough weight and have achieved sufficient muscular development. Otherwise you will find your gains very slow.

There are several additional types of athletics that are also excellent body builders. Wrestling is considered to be the best for all-around body development. Wrestling will develop your physique from head to toe. Most successful wrestlers are also barbell men. They use barbells to increase their strength and muscular development. Gymnastics is recommended to develop the upper part of your body. Any well-equipped gym will have available parallel bars and horizontal bars. Last, but not least, tumbling develops the thighs and calves. You can achieve complete development by combining gymnastics and tumbling. The only drawback to gymnastics is lack of facilities and proper instruction. That is why barbells are the most practical of body builders. They can be used in the home and are convenient for everyone. I would advise parents to encourage their youngsters to take up tennis. Sports such as baseball, football and basketball are soon discarded. But tennis can be played by anyone from ten years of age to eighty. King Gustav of Sweden was still playing tennis at eighty-four. Tennis is wonderful for developing coordination, timing and agility. As of 1975, it is estimated that more than 30 million people are playing tennis in the United States. The parent and child who participate in this sport together become closer. Try it, you'll like it!

Weight training gives the baseball player added power to hit the ball further, and throw harder. In football it increases the player's power both on the line and in the backfield. Weight training strengthens the hands and arms of the basketball player, and makes it difficult for an opponent to "steal" the ball away from him. Many track and field stars find that weight training helps them improve their performance.

The following athletes combined weights with their favorite sports:

The 1974 Superbowl champions, the *Pittsburgh Steelers*, have many members training with weights to strengthen their bodies for the football season. The greatest fear of most athletes is that of being seriously injured. They know that a well-conditioned body will end the season with fewer injuries.

Mercury Morris of the Miami Dolphins is one of the strongest and fastest backs in football. Weight training is an important part of his conditioning program.

Randy White is an outstanding defensive lineman for the Dallas Cowboys. Weight training has helped him become a better and stronger player.

Al Feuerbach, a champion in the shotput, uses weight training to help him break records in this demanding sport.

Brian Oldfield is a fine track-and-field athlete specializing in the discus and the shotput. Weight training has helped him improve his performance.

Bob Seagren, who has broken many records in the pole vault, uses weight training to aid him in his chosen sport.

Advanced course—the set system

You may find, after six months of training with the average course, that your gains have ceased. This means that your body has become accustomed to the exercise and requires a change of routine. In order to make the body respond to further change, you must adopt an advanced course like the set system. Before you begin this new course, take one or two weeks vacation from your former program. Then, your body will be ready.

The set system is nothing more than a special method of repeating the same exercise after a few minutes rest. If you repeat the exercise twice it is a two set system, if you repeat three times it is a three set system. The purpose of the set system is to keep flushing the muscles with blood, thereby increasing its size. The two-arm curl (see page 104) is an example of how this works. After you have completed 10 repetitions, your heart has pumped blood to the biceps, swelling them in size. Then, rest a minute, and the volume of blood in your biceps will subside partially. Now, repeat the exercise with equal or less weight; this will send more blood back to the biceps.

Many athletes who adopted the set system have achieved outstanding results. It is recognized as the most effective method of progressive exercise. The set system has been found to increase the size of the muscles more rapidly than the single exercise system.

It is not necessary to repeat your entire exercise routine. Apply the set system as a form of specialization. If your legs and hips require additional exercise, repeat the squats (see pages 108, 109) and leg press (see page 27). If it is your arm that requires more work, repeat the barbell curls (see page 104) for biceps, and bench presses (see pages 110, 111) for triceps.

20

Advanced course—the set system

Follow the two set system for a few months. You may find that two sets will be ample for you. If it is not enough, try the three set system. It is not necessary, as a rule, to go beyond three sets. The exercises are only a means to an end; you need not spend four hours a day on a workout. You can achieve excellent results by working one hour daily, for three alternate days a week.

Some people may find it too strenuous to complete their full routine in the set system. Modify your routine so that you work the upper body one day, and the lower half the next day. In this way you need not feel exhausted at the end of your workout. By exercising your upper body and lower body separately you can exert more strength in your workouts.

How Calisthenics help you

A great many people keep fit through light calisthenic exercise. Anyone interested only in losing weight will find that calisthenic exercise, together with diet, is sufficient. The man of less than average weight can add 5 to 10 pounds with calisthenics because the calisthenic course includes such exercise as dipping and chinning. If these exercises are properly done, you are working against the resistance of your own body. When you use weights of any kind, be it live weight (such as your body) or dead weights (such as barbells or dumbbells), the exercise becomes a muscle builder. That is precisely where the gain in body weight takes place. Chinning develops the latissimus dorsi muscles (upper back). When these muscles are fully developed, they add considerable weight to your upper body.

If your interest in body building goes no further than calisthenics, you will find that you can keep in good condition and still develop a fairly good physique. Calisthenics, however, cannot build up the legs, hips and the lower back muscle, (the largest mass of muscle in the body) to the fullest extent. These require more resistance to achieve maximum development. The best way to develop them would be with barbells.

There are people who lead an active life and can only find time to take a light calisthenic workout. For them, three valuable exercises are recommended to keep them trim and physically fit. The first exercise is the sit-up for the upper abdominals, and the leg-raise for the lower abdominals (see pages 42, 43). This is the most important of all the exercises; as long as your abdominal muscles are firm you will always be in good shape.

The second exercise is the floor push-up or dip (see page 52). This develops the triceps, or the back of the arm, and the pectorals, or chest muscles (see page 34).

The third is chinning, which develops the latissimus dorsi muscles, or upper back, and the biceps, or front part of arm (see page 48). If you have more time to devote to your workout, try to complete all the calisthenic exercises listed in the book.

Three exercises are recommended for the overweight. These should be performed every day. The first is the sit-up for the upper abdominals, and the leg-raise for the lower abdominals (see pages 42, 43). The second is the side-bend (see page 49). The third is the deep knee-bend for the hips and thighs (see page 44). These exercises should start with 5 repetitions and gradually be worked up to 15 or 20. If you have enough time for a complete workout, you will derive more benefit from it.

A devotee of light exercise may be under the impression that weight training will make him muscle-bound. This is not true. Many athletes, amateurs and professionals, who have trained with weights have succeeded in their chosen sport. Angelo Trulio of New York, who won the 1946 National Four Wall Handball Championship, was a former weight lifting star.

Frank Stranahan of Toledo, Ohio, who won several amateur golf championships, exercised with weights. Handball and golf call for speed, skill and accuracy. These men reached the top of their competitive sports, yet weight training did not interfere with their game.

In football, a great many coaches favor weights because this type of training gives the players more strength and power. Exercise with weights will also help you in your chosen sport.

In one respect, training for physical development is similar to the training for mental development. You cannot remain in the same class, at school, year in and year out. You must advance from the first stage to a higher stage. Calisthenics is the first stage in exercise. If you are to make progress and further develop your body, you must advance from calisthenics to barbells, dumbbells and pulleys.

Chapter 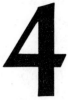 4

Important muscles of the body

THERE ARE certain muscles of the body that should be given more attention than others because they improve your appearance and give you more strength. In this chapter, we will discuss these muscles, their function, and which of the exercises are best suited to build them up.

Deltoid (shoulders), neck and trapezius muscles

Broad shoulders set off a man's appearance. They give him a look of strength and ruggedness. You may fool some people by wearing a suit with tailored broad shoulders, but you cannot fool them when you wear a bathing suit. The development of shoulder muscles is important because they help us to lift weights and objects overhead. They are also important for sports. In boxing the shoulders are usually the first to tire. In baseball the shoulders play an important part in hitting and throwing. In tennis, handball and basketball the shoulders are in constant use.

The shoulder mass is composed of 3 parts: *the front deltoid, the side deltoid,* and *the back deltoid.* The front deltoid is developed by the following exercises: two-arm press with barbell (pages 102, 103), and the front lateral raise with barbells (page 122) or dumbbells (page 76). The side deltoid is developed by the two-arm press behind neck (page 119), the two-arm dumbbell alternate press (pages 56, 57), and the side lateral raise with dumbbells (page 79), or the pulleys exercise (page 94). The back deltoid is developed by the rowing motion with barbells (page 121), or dumbbells (page 72). You can also develop the back deltoids with the pulleys (page 95). These exercises are sufficient for all-around shoulder development.

Wrestlers generally have the largest and most muscular necks. Their necks receive a considerable amount of exercise from constant bridging and trying to escape from headlocks. You are not required, however, to take up wrestling to develop your neck. The body builder's aim should be to develop his neck in *proper proportion* to the rest of his body. A well-formed muscular neck is fine to look at when it blends with your physique. It can also be ugly when developed out of proportion. The average person who begins a course in weight training will find that as he develops his body his neck will increase a little in size. If you want a well-developed neck, you will have to resort to exercises such as the wrestler's bridge with or without weights (see pages 124, 125), and pulley neck exercises (see pages 90, 91).

The trapezius is a large triangular muscle located in the upper back. The development of this muscle is a must for all body builders and especially those who are round-shouldered. A well-developed trapezius helps keep the shoulders back in proper place. A well-developed trapezius plus proper posture (head high, chest out and stomach in) helps to correct a round-shouldered condition. The following exercises will develop the trapezius muscle: the shoulder shrug with barbells (page 116), with dumbbells (page 69), and the upright rowing exercise (page 118).

The rib-box and pectoral muscles

Most body builders want to develop a large chest. The average person is under the impression that the chest consists only of pectoral muscles. This is only partly true. The main object of the exercises should be to *increase the size of the rib-box*. The development of the pectorals should be secondary. The primary reason for increasing the size of your rib-box is not only for the sake of appearance, but to increase the space for your lungs and other organs in the rib-box, so that they are better able to carry on their functions.

Light exercise, such as calisthenics or light dumbbells, is not enough to expand and enlarge the rib-box. To achieve a larger rib-box, you must increase the demand by your lungs for more oxygen. Enforced breathing that results from strenuous exertion, such as the rapid, deep knee-bend with barbells, swimming underwater, and running the hundred yard dash at top speed will help to increase the size of your rib-box.

The deep knee-bend is important for chest development. This particular exercise should become your favorite. Not only will it develop your chest but it will also increase the size and the strength of your thighs and hips.

The deep knee-bend, when done rapidly, 15 to 20 repetitions with a moderate weight, makes you breathe faster. When you do the exercise, open your mouth wide. Take in all the oxygen you can, and hold it, as you lower into a squat. Stop when your thighs are parallel to the floor; then, exhale as you come to the erect position. Make certain that your back is perfectly upright and not bent over, to avoid straining it.

When you have completed the squatting exercise, use a 20 pound barbell or dumbbell, to do the two-arm pullover (page 110). This is an effective combination for increasing the size of your rib-box.

Now, let us consider the development of the pectoral muscles. The pectoral muscles are fairly large muscles covering almost the entire chest. The chief function of the pectoral muscles is to draw the arms forward, downward and across the chest. In order to obtain a full development of these muscles we must practice a variety of exercises, such as the bench press with dumbbells (page 70) and barbells (pages 110, 111), dip on parallel bars, dip on floor (page 52), dip between chairs (page 53), lateral bench press with dumbbells (page 71) and pulleys (page 97).

The dip on parallel bars will develop the lower part of the pectorals. This particular exercise is, in my opinion, the best combination exercise for the pectoral and tricep muscles. This exercise is not included in the apparatus courses, but it should be part of your routine if parallel bars are available.

The pulleys are excellent for all-around development of the pectorals. If you are unable to work with pulleys, you will find the bench press with barbells (pages 110, 111), lateral bench press with dumbbells (page 71), and a variety of floor push-ups and dips on parallel bars, enough to fully develop the pectoral muscles.

Thighs, hips and calves

The thighs and hips are the largest and the most powerful muscles of the body. A strong, well-developed pair of legs is not only pleasing to look at, but a necessity because these muscles carry us through life. First signs of advancing age are felt in the legs. The professional athlete, like the boxer, or baseball player, usually lasts as long as his legs remain in good condition. Many professional athletes are compelled to give up their profession because their legs have lost their speed and power. Every normal person is very much dependent upon his limbs in nearly everything he does, whether it be work or recreation. There is an old saying, "You are as young as you feel." And you will feel younger, more alive and full of pep if your legs are kept in good condition by the correct progressive exercise, like the deep knee-bend, leg pressing machine, and rise-on-toes. These exercises not only develop your thighs, hips and calves, but they will also increase the size of your rib-box. The deep knee-bend with barbells is a strenuous but highly beneficial exercise. After you perform this exercise your breathing will become more pronounced, and you will be forced to inhale more oxygen. This enforced breathing will increase the size of your rib-box.

The deep knee-bend, or squat, is also beneficial for those who want to gain weight. Many body builders have gained anywhere from 10 to 70 pounds, emphasizing this exercise. The thighs and hips are the largest mass of muscle in the body, and we can easily understand why there is an increase in body weight when they are developed and increased in size.

The deep knee-bend is one of the exercises that give you strength, power and energy. If you have a tendency to be underweight, the squat will not only put muscles on your thighs and hips, but it will also help you keep the weight after you have gained it. I have observed that those of my pupils who have gained weight through the deep knee-bend, and later discarded this exercise, find that they suffer a loss of body weight.

There are those who discontinue the deep knee-bend because they may have experienced a strained back, or because they may have poor balance while squatting. Poor balance can be overcome by putting a one or two inch block of wood under your heels.

Although weight training is recognized as the best medium for body building, certain hazards do exist. They can, however, be easily avoided if simple precautions are taken in exercises like the dead lift or the deep knee-bend.

Some weight training instructors advise full, deep knee-bend for best results. By full, deep knee-bend, we mean that the buttocks are nearly touching the floor. There are others who believe in the half-squat; that is, with the thighs parallel to the floor. I favor the half-squat because there is less danger of straining your lower back.

If you train at home by yourself, it is advisable to obtain a

Important muscles of the body

pair of deep knee-bending stands, shown in Fig. 133, page 109. If you do the deep knee-bend with barbell weights of 150 pounds or more, without these stands, too much energy is spent lifting the weight and placing it behind your head. When you have completed the squatting exercise, you will find it much easier to place the weight on the stands, than lifting the weight overhead and returning it to the floor.

There are some body builders who use as much as 300 to 400 pounds in a deep knee-bend. This is not necessary. You can gradually work up to using weights that range from 150 to 250 pounds and develop a pair of strong, well-developed thighs in the process.

The leg pressing machine is a good substitute exercise for the deep knee-bend, and will definitely take the strain off the back. This type of apparatus is usually found in a gymnasium. The weights are loaded on a small raised platform. You lie on your back below the platform, and place your feet up against the bottom of the platform. "Press up" the weighted platform with your legs, until your legs are fully extended. You will find that you can add more weight with the leg pressing machine than with the deep knee-bend, because the back is not being used in this exercise. It is essentially a thigh and hip movement.

The calves are the most difficult of all muscles to increase in size because they are constantly used for walking. Walking does not give calves the full contraction that you would receive from running, climbing steps, and rising on toes. To build calf muscles, we emphasize the rise-on-toes. There are three different ways to do this exercise: toes pointed in, toes pointed out, and toes pointed straight (see pages 46, 120).

If you should find that your calves do not respond, or have stopped growing, try doing your calf raises with weights on your back (see page 120), or with dumbbell in your hand. For best results, rise on your toes as high as possible.

The latissimus dorsi and erector spinal muscles

The important back muscles we are interested in are the latissimus dorsi and erector spinal muscles (see page 34).

The latissimus dorsi is a large, fan-shaped, triangular muscle. Most body builders are interested in developing this muscle because of the pleasing appearance it gives them, and because it is one of the easiest muscles to develop. The latissimus dorsi muscle, when fully developed, will make your back very broad. The function of this muscle is to lower the arms and move them back. There are three types of exercises used to develop the latissimus dorsi muscles: chinning (page 48), rowing motion (page 121) and pulleys (page 86), and the latissimus dorsi machine, an advanced pulley exercise machine expressly made to exercise the latissimus dorsi muscle.

Chinning is the simplest, and one of the favorite exercises of most body builders. It is also my opinion that this is the most effective way to develop the latissimus dorsi muscles, and it should be high on your list.

There are various methods used in chinning. The most popular is chinning with the underhand grip, shoulder width apart (page 48). There is also the backhand chin. Here, the backs of your hands face you as you grasp the bar. You draw yourself up and bring your chin over the bar. Another method is the back-of-the-neck chin. Grasp the bar with the overhand grip, more than shoulder width apart. Draw yourself up and forward, so that the back of your neck touches the bar. Finally, there is the advanced chin, done with weights. Attach a line rope with a weight around your hips. A 10 to 20 pound weight is satisfactory. If you can, do 10 or more repetitions with it. If you increase your repetitions to 15, add 5 to 10 pounds, and begin over again with 10 repetitions.

When you chin, be sure to do a *complete* movement. Your chin should be raised up over the bar, and when you return to the hanging position your arms should be fully extended (page 48).

There are several good substitutes for those who cannot chin, because they are overweight or too weak to chin more than 2 or 3 times. The overweight should use the pulleys (page 86), rowing exercise with barbells (page 121) or the dumbbells (page 72). They should perform enough repetitions to lose weight. 20 to 30 repetitions should be sufficient. If you are underweight and find chinning too difficult, do as many chins as you can, and then perform the rowing motion with barbells.

We now come to the erector spinal muscles (see page 35). These muscles may not look as spectacular as the latissimus dorsi; however, they are more important to the proper function of your back. The erector spinal muscles resemble two large cables. They are located in the center of the lower back, and help support the spine and vertebrae.

Important muscles of the body

The erector spinal muscles, when fully developed, help cushion the back against shocks and strains. A great many people suffer from back trouble because of the lack of proper exercise, and they succumb to strains, aches and lumbago from lifting a comparatively light weight. These weaknesses can be eliminated if you build a strong back. A strong back is also absolutely necessary for everybody who wants to go through life feeling healthy and energetic. The dead lift with barbells is one of the best exercises for the lower back muscles (see pages 114, 115) as is the calisthenic back exercise (pages 38, 39).

Caution: When you perform the dead lift with heavy weights, *keep the knees slightly bent at all times.* This reduces the likelihood of straining your back.

Abdomen (stomach muscles) and external oblique (side muscles)

There is a saying that fat men are a happy and jolly lot. I have asked many people who are overweight whether they were contented with their present physical condition. Ninety-nine per cent answered that they felt miserable, carrying around excess fat, and would much rather possess a trim and healthy physique.

Insurance rates are always higher for the overweight. Statistics show that fat people generally succumb to diseases such as high blood pressure, heart trouble and diabetes, all of which cut the life span short. Watch your weight carefully. If you are overweight, see your doctor and have him put you on a diet. Although exercise alone will not remove the fat from your body, it will strengthen and harden your muscles, and the diet will remove the excess weight.

Between the ages of thirty to forty, one usually begins to take on added weight. Fat collects around the abdominal wall because it is the least active muscle. Most people believe that participation in sports like handball, swimming, golf or tennis will develop their stomach muscles. This is far from the truth. You should perform special abdominal exercises such as sit-ups for the upper abdominals, and leg-raises for the lower abdominals, to keep these muscles in good condition.

Since the stomach muscles aid in digestion and elimination, it is essential that you keep them in good shape. It is my opinion that the abdominal muscles are the most important in the body. If you do nothing else but keep your waistline trim and firm, you will always look and feel healthy.

Here's power for you

Two exercise movements are necessary to develop the stomach muscles. The first is the ordinary sit-up (page 42). The second movement develops the lower part of the abdomen (page 43).

The overweight person who has not as yet done any abdominal exercise, should begin with 4 to 5 repetitions according to his ability. If he feels as though his stomach might cramp, he should stop immediately and refrain from doing any more abdominal exercise in this workout period. The next time, he can gradually increase the repetitions by one a week until he reaches a total of 20 repetitions.

The man who wants to *gain* weight should also do the two abdominal exercises, namely, the sit-up with hands clasped behind the head (page 42) and leg-raise (page 43).

Begin with 5 repetitions of each exercise and increase them by one or 2 weekly, depending on the degree of exercise your stomach muscles can stand. When you can perform 15 repetitions in each exercise, you will be ready to do your abdominal exercises described on pages 60, 61, 106, and 107.

The external oblique muscles are commonly known as the side muscles. These, together with the abdominal muscles, should be strengthened through exercise. They help prevent rupture when you lift an awkward or heavy weight. Well-developed side muscles also help you to carry objects greater distances.

The simplest and most effective way to develop these muscles is the side exercise described on pages 49, 77 and 113.

Biceps, triceps and forearms

Almost every body builder wants to develop large muscular biceps, and I am all for it. However, we must remember that there are other muscles to be developed in addition to the biceps; the biceps do not constitute the entire arm. The triceps, for example (see page 35), which makes up the back of the arm, is a three-headed muscle. It is much larger than the biceps which is a two-headed muscle. In all lifts, in which weights are raised overhead from the floor, the biceps play a minor role. The triceps, legs, and back are far more important.

Some individuals will make more rapid gains, developing their arms, than others because of their physical structure. The overweight will probably reach his goal much sooner by reducing, diet and exercise, than the man who is underweight. The slim athlete will also make satisfactory gains by exercising

Important muscles of the body

regularly, sticking to a weight-gaining diet, and getting enough sleep.

The beginner who follows the average course will probably increase the size of his arms within the first six months. If he finds that he is not gaining rapidly enough, he can try specialized training for his arms. He might adopt the set system, described on page 20. For example: he might begin with the two-arm curl with barbells (page 104), repeating the exercise 10 times. Then, he will put the weights down and rest for a minute or two, after which, he repeats the same exercise. Another effective bicep builder is the one-and-a-half curl. Use a weight about 20 pounds lighter than the one ordinarily used in the curl. Curl the weight up to your shoulders. Then, uncurl the weight down slowly until your forearm is straight out and parallel to the floor. Now, curl the weight back to the shoulder. Do one full curl and then one half-curl. The complete exercise requires 10 full curls and 10 half-curls. This type of curl can be done with barbells and dumbbells. It has been proven very satisfactory for specialized and advanced training.

To develop the biceps, the following exercises are used: the two-arm barbell curl (page 104), the two-arm dumbbell curl (page 59), the one-arm bend over dumbbell curl (page 81), and the one-and-a-half barbell or dumbbell curl.

We now come to the triceps. You will achieve large muscular arms only by developing the biceps and the triceps to the fullest extent. The triceps seem to respond more rapidly to exercise than the biceps. I believe the barbell bench press (page 111) is a valuable exercise. Not only does it increase the size of the triceps, but it exercises the shoulders and the pectorals as well. It also helps to develop remarkable strength and power in your arms. This may well become one of your favorite exercises. Both overweight and underweight can benefit from it. When you reach the advanced stage and can do three sets of bench presses with a fairly heavy weight, you will undoubtedly have developed large triceps. Another fine triceps exercise is the dip on parallel bars. In this exercise you must have some degree of strength in order to perform it. If you are a beginner, I suggest that you start with the push-ups on the floor (page 52). This is the simplest form of dip. Begin with about 5 dips, and add one or two each week, until you can perform 20 dips. When you do the push-ups, be sure that your body is kept in a perfectly straight line from head

31

to foot. Bend your arms and lower your body until your chest touches the floor. Then, push up until your arms are fully extended.

In order to obtain the maximum benefit from your exercises, a complete contraction and extention is necessary, that is, you do *full* movements and not *half* motions. When you can perform 20 or 30 push-ups, you will be ready for the dip on parallel bars. When you can accomplish 15 dips on the parallel bars, you will be ready for the advanced dip with weights. To increase the resistance and to make this exercise more effective, do the dip on parallel bars, supporting weights. You will need a piece of rope and a weight of 10 pounds. Tie the rope around your hips with the 10 pound weight suspended between your thighs. Then, do your dips.

The following exercises will also develop the triceps: two-arm press with barbells (pages 102, 103), two-arm press behind neck with barbells (page 119), two-arm alternate dumbbell press (pages 56, 57), and one-arm dumbbell press (pages 74, 75). You will be able to achieve good results with these exercises.

If the beginner concentrates on the larger muscles of the body, the forearms will receive enough exercise during these workouts. After you have obtained a reasonably well-developed physique, you may want to increase the size of your forearms. You will find that as your forearms increase in strength and size, your wrists will also develop. The forearms, like the calves, are difficult to develop because forearm muscles are used continuously in our daily work. Don't give up if you find it difficult to develop the forearms. There are special exercises for this purpose. They should be done while seated on a bench. Place a 20 pound dumbbell or barbell over your knees, using an underhand grip. Bend your wrist down as far as it will go. Now, bring the weight forward by flexing your wrists. Continue this for 10 repetitions. When you can complete 15 repetitions, add 5 pounds and begin over again with 10 repetitions. The next exercise is the same as the first, but the movements are reversed. Use an overhand grip, and flex wrists up and down. The following exercise can only be done with dumbbells. Hold both dumbbells over your knees and rotate them from side to side.

This chart indicates which of the exercises (calisthentics, dumbbells, pulleys or barbells) will build up the individual muscles of the body.

MUSCLES	CALISTHENICS	DUMBBELLS	PULLEYS	BARBELLS
Neck	Resist ex., p. 40, 41	Wrestler's bridge, p. 82	Neck ex., p. 90, 91	Wrestler's bridge, p. 124
Trapezius		Shoulder shrug, p. 69		Shoulder shrug, p. 116 / Upright rowing, p. 118
Pectorals	Push-ups, p. 52, 53	Lat. bench press, p. 71 / 2-arm alt. bench press, p. 70	Pectoral ex., p. 97	Bench press, p. 111
Deltoids		2-arm alt. press, p. 56 / 2-arm alt. bench press, p. 70 / 1-arm press, p. 74 / Front lat. raise, p. 76 / Back deltoid ex., p. 78 / Side lat. raise, p. 79	1-arm front lat. raise, p. 93 / 1-arm side lat. raise, p. 94	2-arm press, p. 102 / Press behind neck, p. 119 / Front lat. raise (stdg.) p. 122
Rib-box		2-arm pull-over, p. 65		2-arm pull-over, p. 110
Triceps	Push-ups, p. 52, 53	2-arm alt. press, p. 56 / 2-arm alt. bench press, p. 70	Triceps ex., p. 96 / 2-arm press, p. 87	2-arm press, p. 102 / Bench press, p. 111 / Press behind neck, p. 119
Biceps	Chinning, p. 48 / Bicep ex., p. 54	2-arm alt. curl, p. 59 / Bend over 1-arm curl, p. 81	Bicep ex., p. 88, 89	2-arm curl, p. 104
Latissimus Dorsi	Chinning, p. 48	1-arm rowing, p. 72	Latissimus dorsi ex., p. 86	Rowing motion, p. 121
Erector Spinal	Back ex., p. 38, 39	Dead weight lift, p. 66, 67		Dead weight lift, p. 115
Abdominals	Sit-ups, p. 42 / Leg-raise, p. 43	Sit-ups, p. 60 / Leg raise, p. 61		Sit-ups, p. 106 / Leg-raise, p. 107
Hips	Knee-bend, p. 44 / Hip ex., p. 50	Knee-bend, p. 64		Knee-bend, p. 108
Thighs	Knee-bend, p. 44, 45	Knee-bend, p. 64		Knee-bend, p. 108
Calves	Rise-on-toes, p. 46			Rise-on-toes, p. 120
Forearms, wrists	Forearms, ex., p. 32			

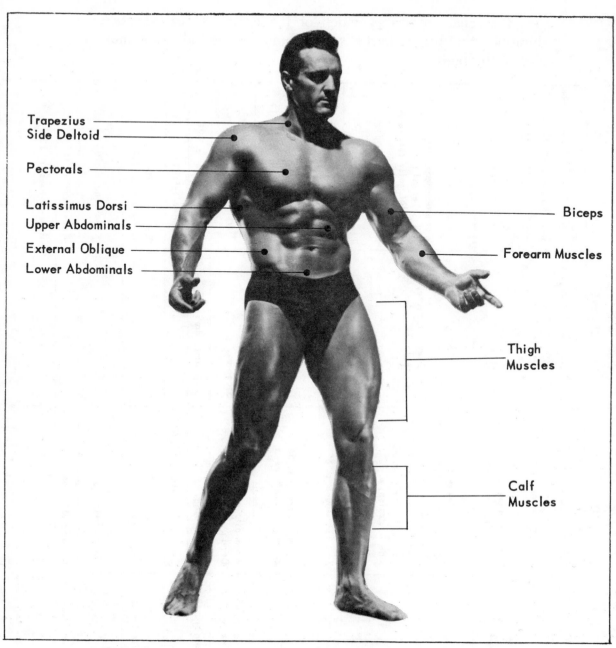

Trapezius
Side Deltoid
Pectorals
Latissimus Dorsi
Upper Abdominals
External Oblique
Lower Abdominals

Biceps
Forearm Muscles
Thigh Muscles
Calf Muscles

Fig. 2   Photo of Clarence Ross, Alameda, Calif.

The front and back view photographs on these pages illustrate the important muscles of the body, referred to in the training guide chart on page 33. Try to familiarize yourself with the names of the muscles. This will make it easier for you to follow the text and the exercise instructions.

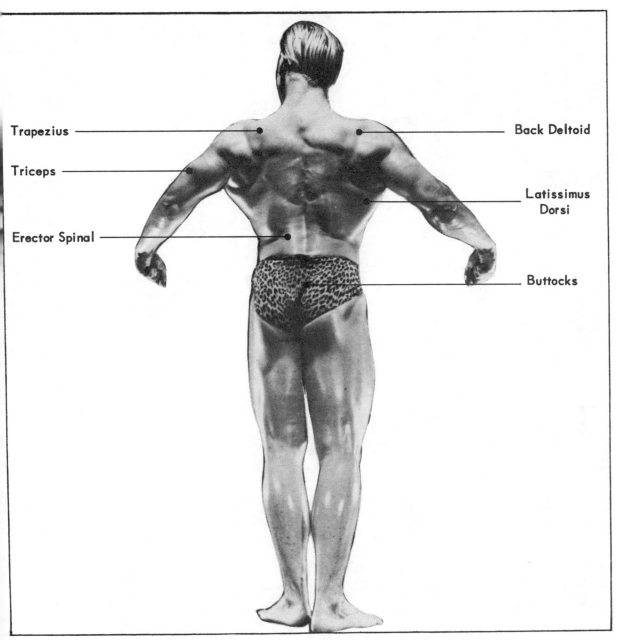

Trapezius

Triceps

Erector Spinal

Back Deltoid

Latissimus Dorsi

Buttocks

Fig. 3   Photo of Al Stephan, Minneapolis, Minn.

If you are not completely familiar with the names of the muscles, it may be necessary to refer back to these photographs from time to time. You might slip a book mark between these pages to make it easier to find, as you read the book.

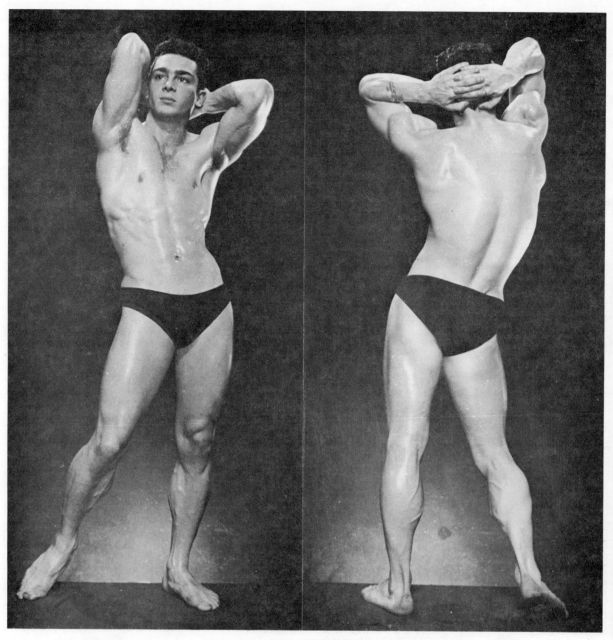

Fig. 4 Photo by Jack Sidney, Brooklyn, New York

Jack Mercury (*Fig. 4* and *Fig. 5*) is an excellent example of what can be achieved mainly through well planned calisthenics exercises. Although not heavily muscled, he has succeeded in building up sinewy, powerful, well-defined muscles and a well-proportioned body. Jack Mercury stands 5 feet 6 inches tall and weighs 145 pounds.

Chapter 5

Calisthenics
Exercise Course

THE FOLLOWING calisthenics course can do more than keep you physically fit. The chinning exercise (page 48) develops the latissimus dorsi muscles, the advanced knee-bend (page 45) increases the strength and size of your thigh muscles, and the advanced push-ups (page 53) add bulk and power to your triceps and pectoral muscles.

Donald Simon, the model for the calisthenics course, is a slender, well-proportioned boy of 15—an excellent example of proper physical development for his years, with great promise for the future.

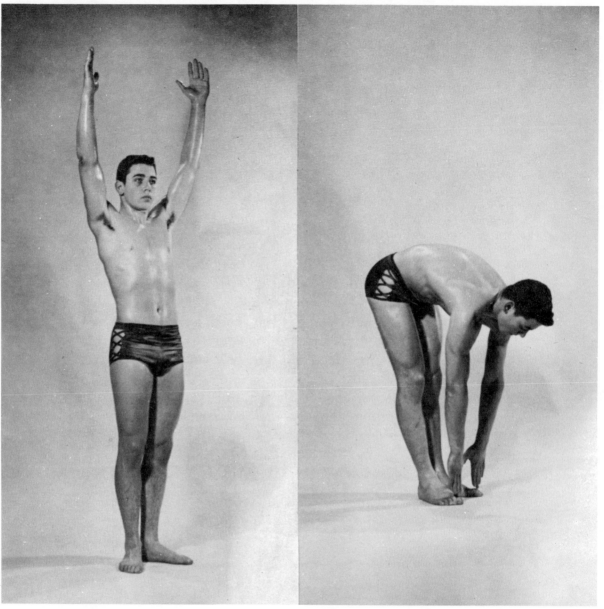

Fig. 6   Fig. 7

Stand erect, arms at your sides, feet close together. Inhale and stretch your arms overhead as high as they will go (*Fig. 6*). Bend over, exhale, and touch your toes (*Fig. 7*), keeping your knees straight. Then, return to original position. Repeat 10 times. After two weeks of continued exercise, add one bend each week until you reach a total of 15 repetitions.

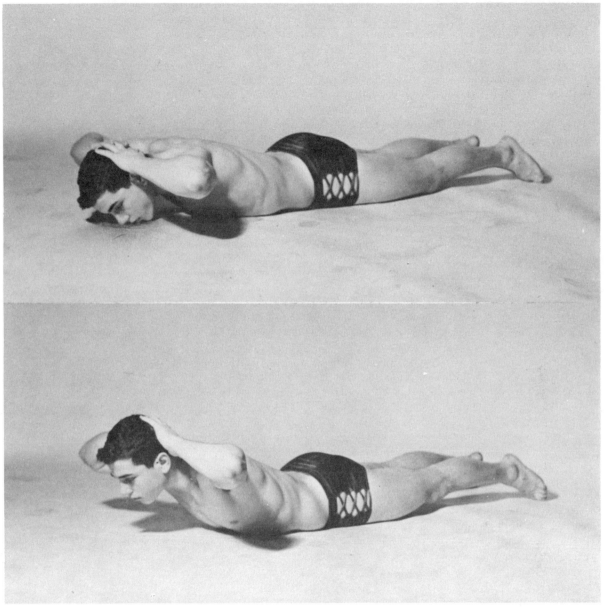

Fig. 8 (upper)   Fig. 9 (lower)

For more advanced exercise to develop lower back muscles, lie with your stomach flat on floor, hands clasped behind your head (*Fig. 8*). From this position, raise your head and body up from the floor (*Fig. 9*), inhaling as you go up and exhaling as you lower your body. Repeat 5 times. After one week, add one movement each week until you reach 15. To get the most out of this exercise, have someone hold your ankles down, or place a heavy object over them.

39

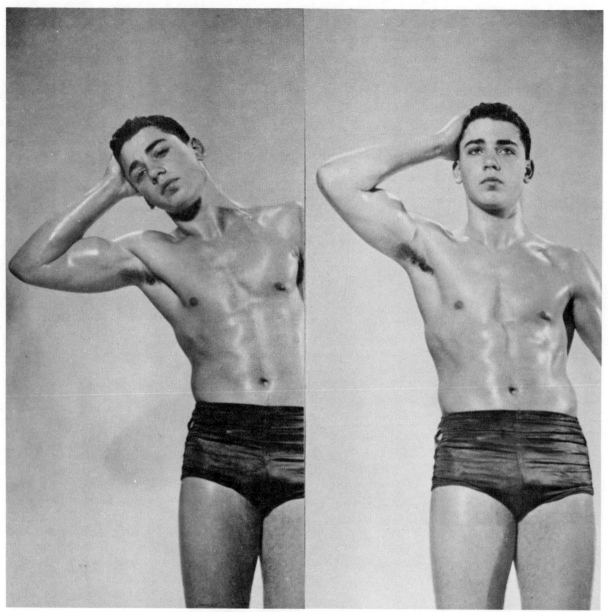

Fig. 10   Fig. 11

   Move the right side of your head close to your right shoulder. Place your right hand against the right side of your head (*Fig. 10*). Push your head toward your left shoulder (*Fig. 11*), resisting with your head. Now, reverse the procedure. Bring the left side of your head close to your left shoulder. Place your left hand against the left side of your head, and push your head toward your right shoulder.

40

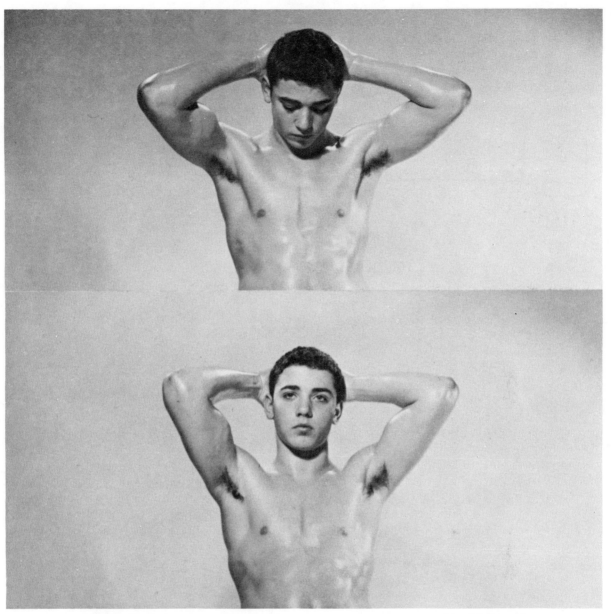

Fig. 12 (upper)   Fig. 13 (lower)

For the next exercise, lower your head to your chest. Clasp both hands behind your head (*Fig. 12*) and force it back to an erect position (*Fig. 13*), resisting with your clasped hands. Reverse the exercise: bend your head back and clasp your hands behind your head. Push forward with your hands (*Fig. 13*), resisting with your head, until your chin touches your chest (*Fig. 12*). Repeat each exercise 10 times. After 1 week, add one repetition each week until you reach 15.

41

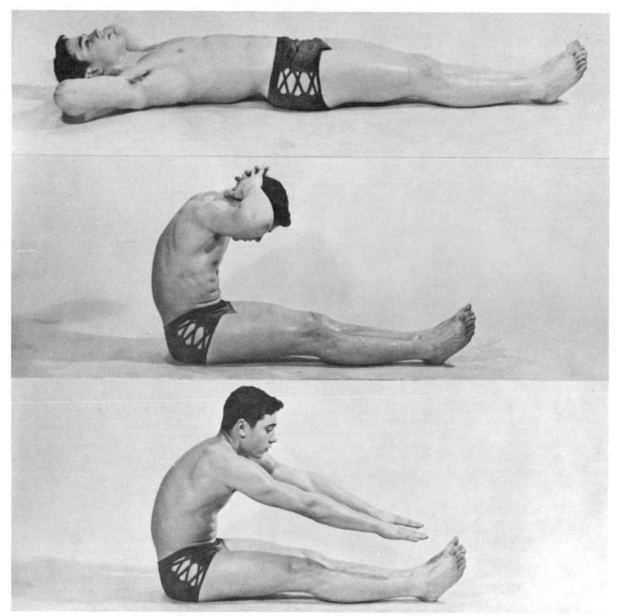

Fig. 14 (upper)   Fig. 15 (middle)   Fig. 16 (lower)

Lie on the floor. Clasp hands behind head (*Fig. 14*). Take a deep breath, and sit up, exhaling as you go up (*Fig. 15*). Then, extend palms to toes (*Fig. 16*). Inhale as you return to original position (*Fig. 15*). The overweight, who have difficulty, should place their hands straight out in front of them at arms length. This enables them to swing forward more easily. You may need a heavy object to hold your feet in place as you raise and lower your body.

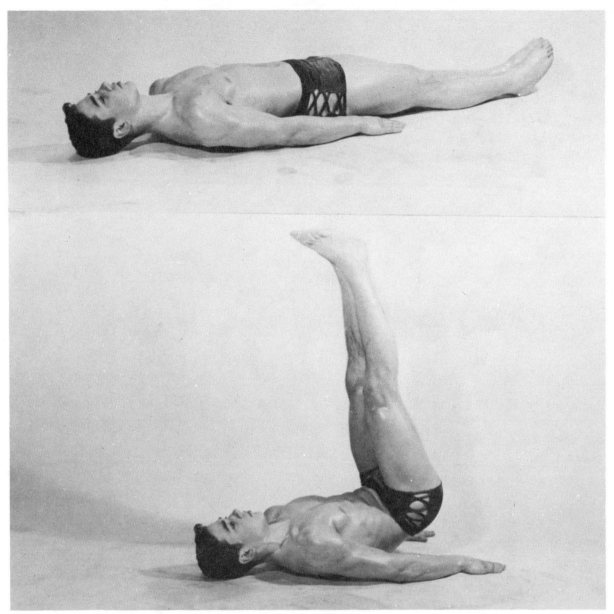

Fig. 17 (upper)   Fig. 18 (lower)

For the lower abdominals, assume position in *Fig. 17*, hands next to sides, palms touching the floor. Take a deep breath and raise both feet to a 90° (*Fig. 18*). Lower legs to floor and exhale. Keep legs straight throughout the exercise. Repeat both exercises 5 times. After several weeks, add one repetition each week until you reach 15. If you cannot raise your legs straight up, raise both knees back to your chest, and then back to floor.

43

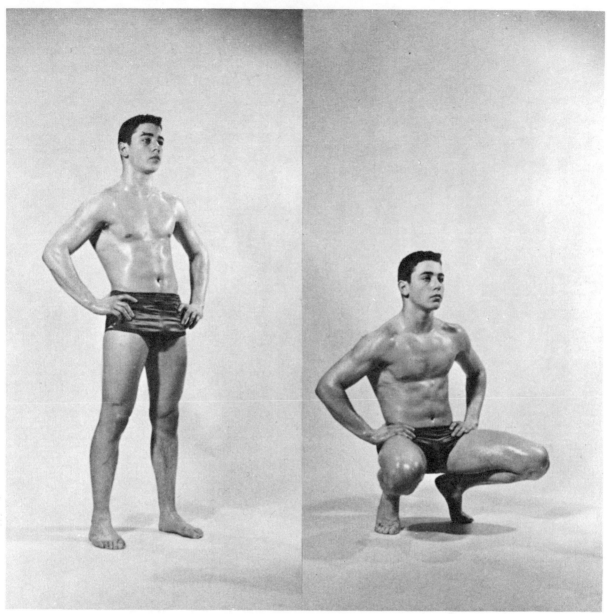

Fig. 19   Fig. 20

Place both hands on your hips (*Fig. 19*), take a deep breath, and lower your body, keeping your back straight (*Fig. 20*). Then, return to the original position, and exhale. Repeat this exercise 10 times. After a week, add 2 bends each week until you reach a total of 20.

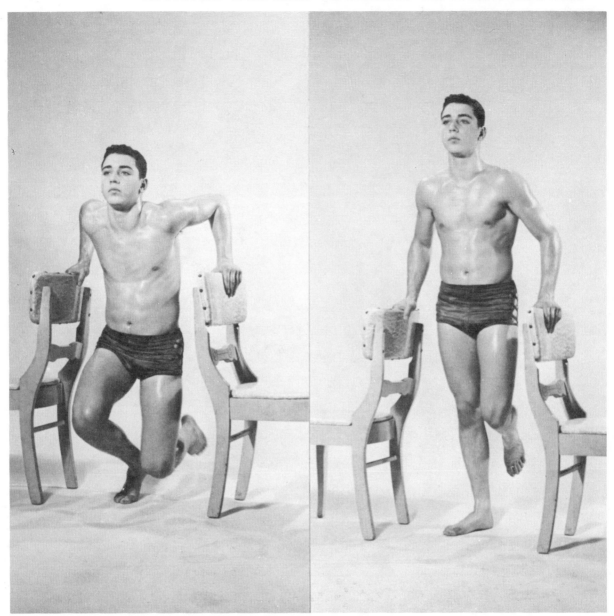

Fig. 21   Fig. 22

After two months, you will be ready for the advanced deep knee-bend. Stand between two chairs, and grasp the backs. Fold your left leg up, inhale, and bend your right leg into a half-squat position (*Fig. 21*). Now, resting on your right leg, raise your body to an upright position (*Fig. 22*), and exhale. Perform the same exercise with the position of your legs reversed. Repeat 5 times. After two weeks, add one movement each week until you reach 10.

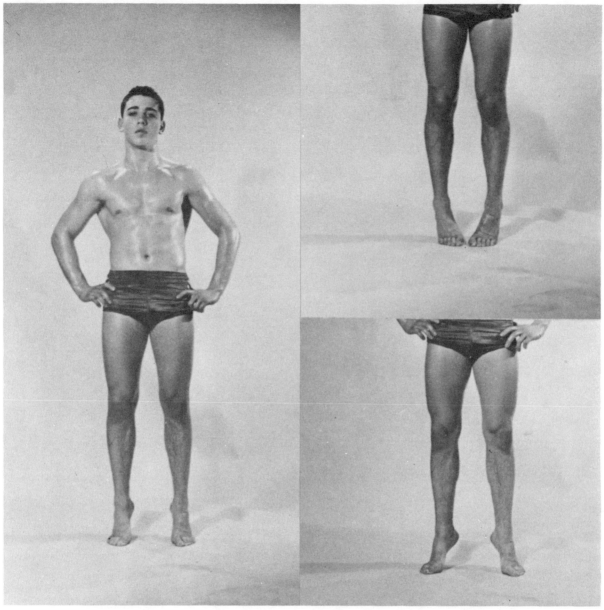

Fig. 23   Fig. 24 (upper)   Fig. 25 (lower)

Place your hands on hips, feet parallel to each other. Rise on your toes as high as you can go (*Fig. 23*). Then, lower your heels to the floor. Now, do the same exercise with toes pointed in (*Fig. 24*), and toes pointed out (*Fig. 25*). Repeat each of the three calf exercises 10 times. After one week, add one repetition a week until you reach a total of 15.

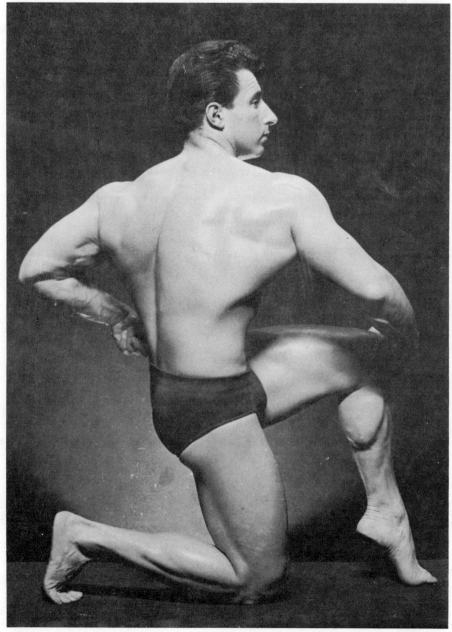

Fig. 26

This photo of Edward Giuliani shows well-developed latissimus dorsi muscles. Chinning (page 48) is an effective exercise
for these muscles. The one-arm rowing exercise with dumbbells
(page 72) and the pulley exercise (page 86) are also good. For
additional development, see rowing exercise with barbells (page
121).

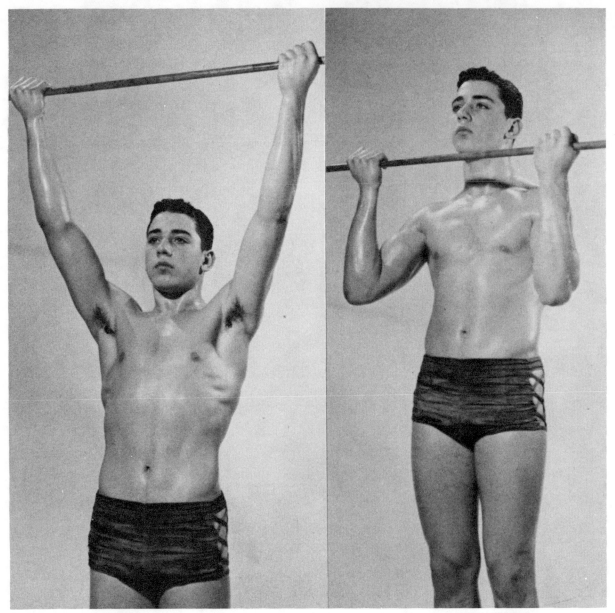

Fig. 27   Fig. 28

Grasp the bar about shoulder width apart, your arms fully extended (*Fig. 27*). Take a deep breath and raise your body until your chin is over the bar (*Fig. 28*). Return to original position and exhale. Try to do this exercise 10 times. After several weeks, add one repetition each week until you reach 15. If you cannot chin 10 times, do as many as you can for several weeks. Then, try to add one to your repetitions each week.

48

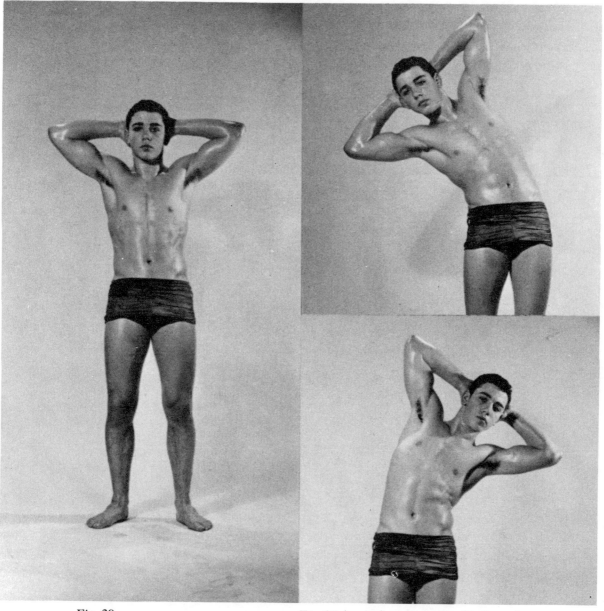

Fig. 29   Fig. 30 (upper)   Fig. 31 (lower)

Stand erect, feet about 12 inches apart, hands clasped behind your head (*Fig. 29*). With one continuous motion, bend your
body sideways to the right as far as it will go (*Fig. 30*), and
then far over to the left side (*Fig. 31*). From this position, swing
back again to the right side (*Fig. 30*). Repeat this exercise 10
times. After several weeks, add one movement each week until
you reach a total of 15.

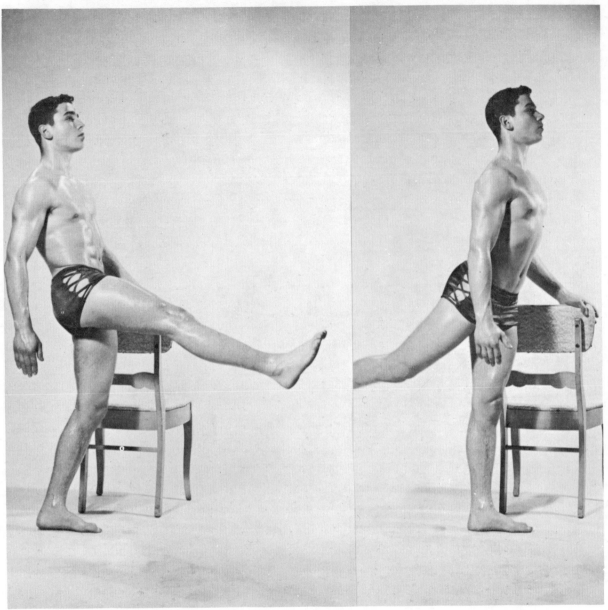

Fig. 32   Fig. 33

Stand alongside a chair and grasp the top with your left hand. Swing your right leg forward as high as you can (*Fig. 32*), and then back as far as it will go (*Fig. 33*). Do exercise as one continuous movement: forward and back. Change position and grasp the chair with your right hand. Now, repeat the exercise by swinging your left leg. Perform exercise 10 times with each leg. After the first week, add one repetition each week until you reach 15.

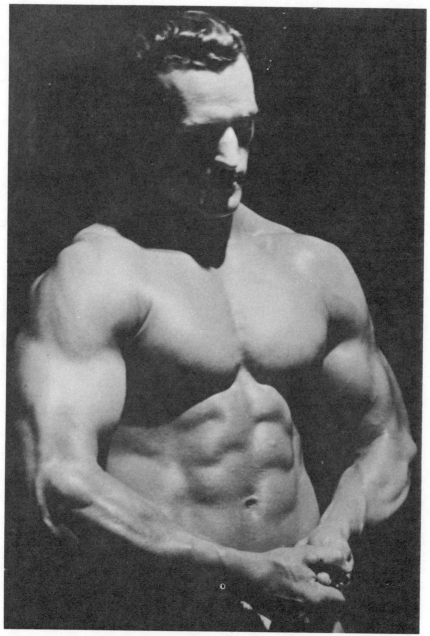

Fig. 34   Photo courtesy of Weider Publications, Jersey City, N. J.

Clarence "Clancy" Ross demonstrates highly developed pectoral and tricep muscles. The push-ups on page 52 is an excellent way to get started. Mr. Ross possesses one of the finest physiques in the country. Among the many awards that he has won are "Mr. America," "Mr. U.S.A.," "Mr. North America," and "Professional Mr. America." He now operates a successful gym in Alameda, California.

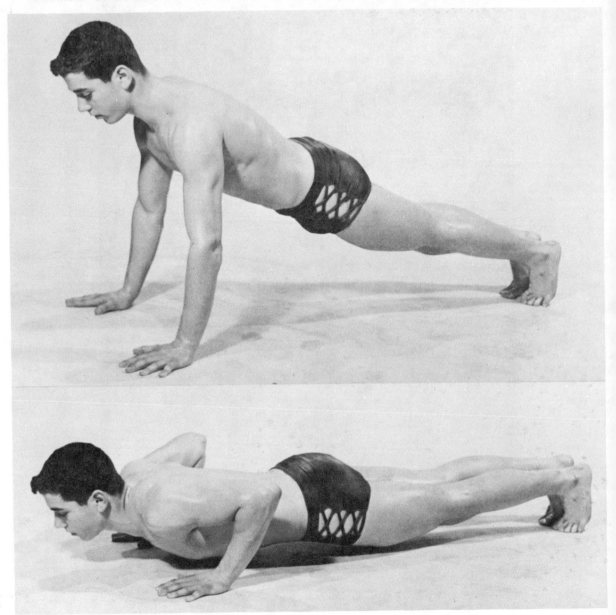

Fig. 35 (upper)   Fig. 36 (lower)

Assume position in *Fig. 35*. Your weight is supported by the palms of your hands and toes. Your body is held in a straight line. Take a deep breath, bend your arms, and lower your body until your chest almost touches the floor (*Fig. 36*). Now, push back to starting position, and exhale. Begin with 5 to 10 repetitions. After several weeks, add one dip each week until you reach a total of 15.

52

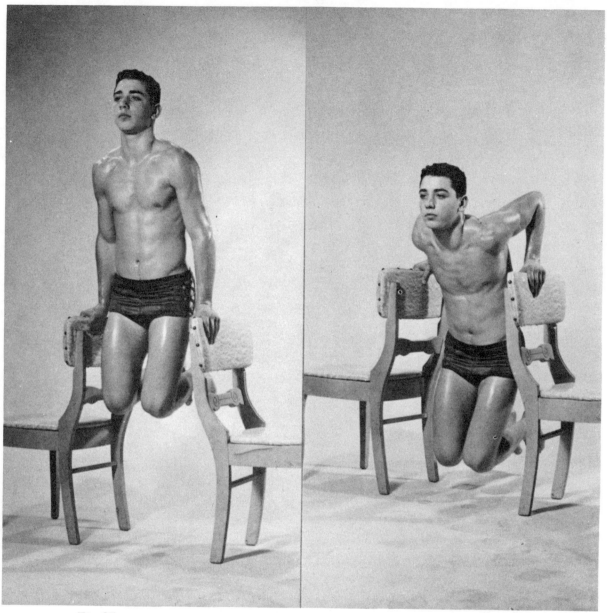

Fig. 37

Fig. 38

Before you try advanced dipping, you should be capable of 30 floor dips without difficulty. Stand between two chairs, grasping the top of each chair. Raise your body until your arms are fully extended, with your feet tucked under you (*Fig. 37*). Then, take a deep breath and dip down as far as you can go, with your feet curled up as in *Fig. 38*. Now, return to original position and exhale. Repeat 5 times. After 2 weeks, add one repetition a week until you reach 10.

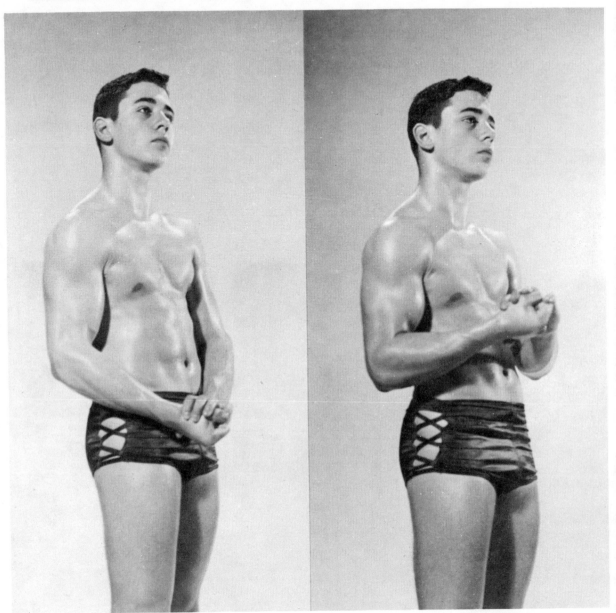

Fig. 39   Fig. 40

Clench the fist of your right hand with your arm extended straight down at your side. Now, grasp your right fist with your left hand and, resisting with your left hand, raise your right hand towards your shoulder (*Figs. 39, 40*). Return to the original position and perform the exercise with your left arm. Repeat 10 times. After the first week, add one each week until you reach 15.

Chapter 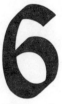 6

Dumbbell
Exercise Course

WHEN YOU are confined to an area, too small for barbell work, you will find that exercising with dumbbells is an effective way to build up your body. (The best type of dumbbells are the plate-loading bells, rather than the solid dumbbells. These permit you to add exact weight to the dumbbells as you require it.)

The models for this chapter are Scott Suretsky and Jed Kaminetsky. Scott has been working out with dumbells and barbells for several years. His photos have appeared in body building magazines. Jed is a promising young athlete who used dumbells and barbells to improve his athletic performance.

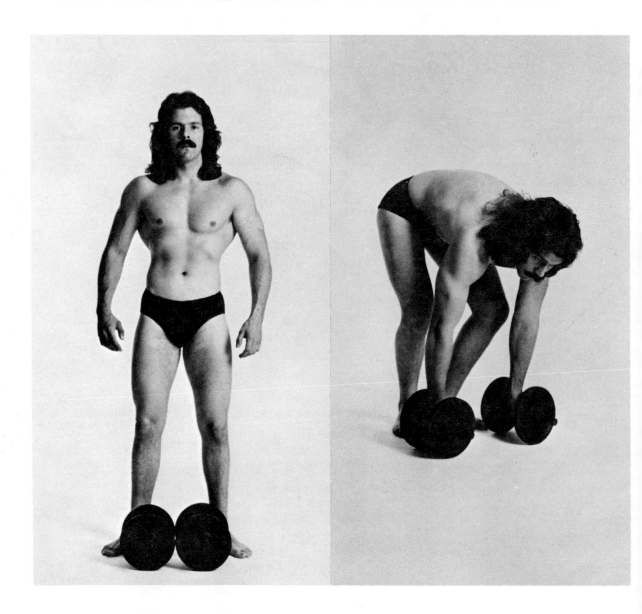

Fig. 41   Fig. 42

Stand erect, your feet about 12 inches apart, with 15 or 20 pound dumbbells in front of you (*Fig. 41*). Bend your knees, lower your body, and grasp the dumbbells (*Fig. 42*). Then, lift both dumbbells to your shoulders with a quick heave (*Fig. 43*). Now, press left dumbbell overhead (*Fig. 44*), inhaling as you go up. Exhale as you lower it back to your shoulder, and raise your right dumbbell overhead, alternating the movements with

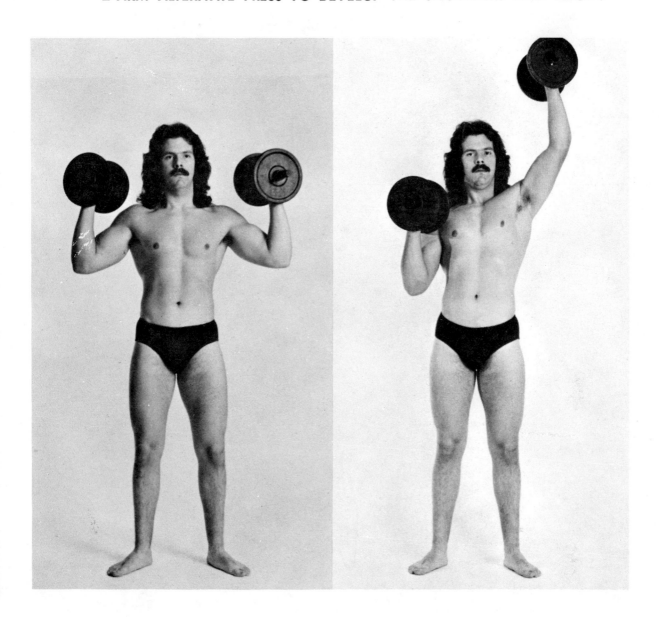

Fig. 43   Fig. 44

each hand. Repeat 10 times with each arm. After several weeks, add one movement each week until you reach 15. For additional development, add 5 pounds to each dumbbell and begin again with 10 repetitions. This exercise can also be done by pressing both dumbbells overhead at the same time, in one movement.

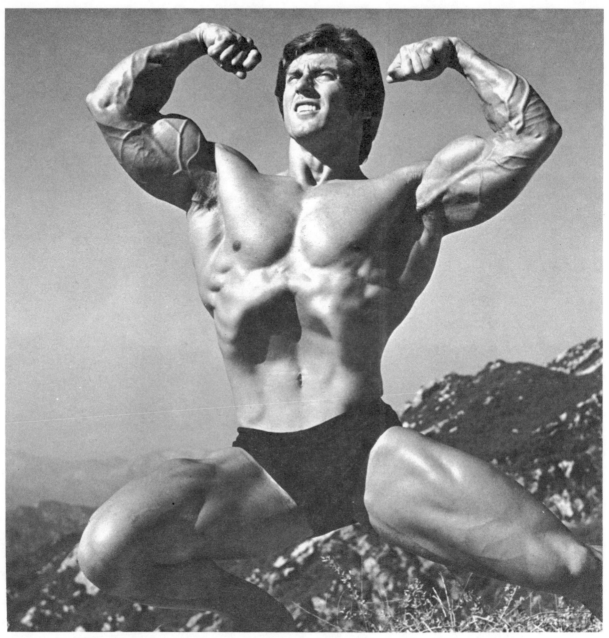

Fig. 45   Photo by Art Zeller, Santa Monica, Ca.

Here is a goal to shoot at for biceps development. The two-arm dumbbell curl (page 59) produces good results. The two-arm barbell curl (page 104) and pulley curls (pages 88, 89) will also add power and size to your biceps. Frank Zane has been awarded the "Mr. America" and "Mr. Universe" titles.

58

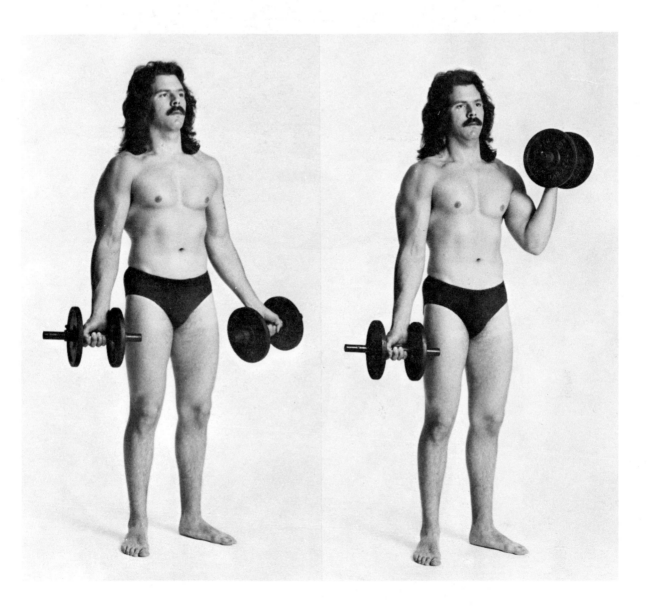

Fig. 46   Fig. 47

Hold a 15 or 20 pound dumbbell in each hand, alongside your body (*Fig. 46*). Curl the dumbbell in your left hand slowly to your shoulder (*Fig. 47*), inhaling as you go up. As you lower it, exhale and curl the dumbbell in your right hand slowly to your shoulder. Repeat 10 times. After several weeks, add one movement each week until you reach 15. For further development, add 5 pounds to each dumbbell and begin with 10 repetitions.

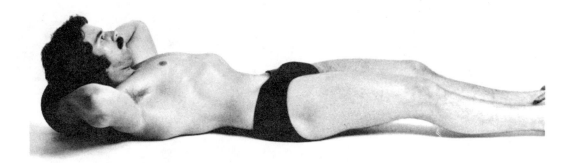

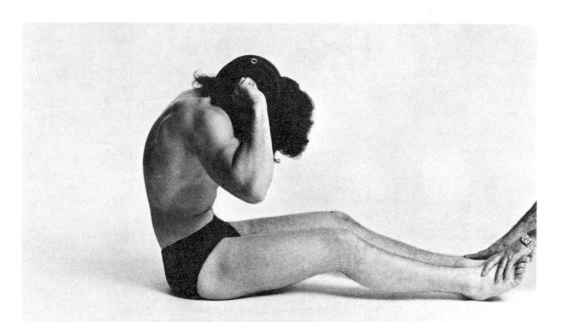

Fig. 48 (upper)   Fig. 49 (lower)

After two months of calisthenic abdominal exercises, you are ready to sit up with weights. Begin with a 5 pound dumbbell. Lie on your back. Place feet below a heavy, stationary object, or, have someone hold them in place. Hold dumbbell behind your head (*Fig. 48*), take a deep breath, and sit up (*Fig. 49*), exhaling as you go. Now, lower your back slowly to floor. Repeat 10 times. After several weeks, add one repetition each week until you reach 15. Then add 2½ pounds and return to 10 repetitions.

60

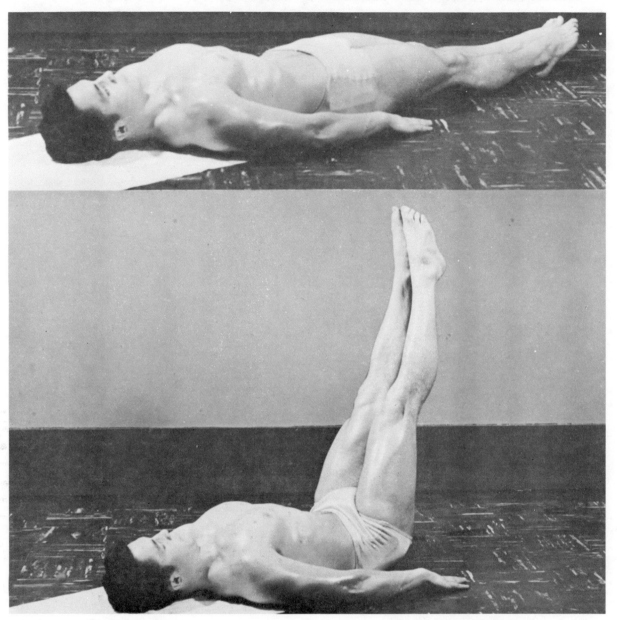

Fig. 50 (upper)   Fig. 51 (lower)

To exercise the lower abdominals, assume position in *Fig. 50*, hands next to sides, palms touching the floor. Take a deep breath and raise both feet to a 90° angle (*Fig. 51*). Lower legs back to floor, and exhale. Keep legs straight throughout the exercise. Repeat 5 times. After several weeks add one repetition each week, until you reach 15.

61

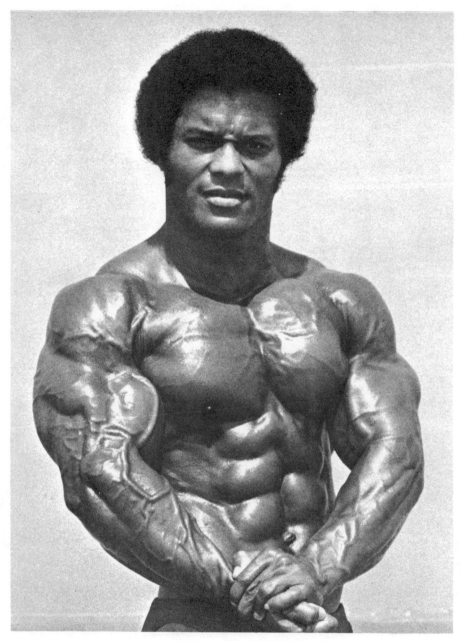

Fig. 52   Photo by Art Zeller, Santa Monica, Ca.

This photo of Ricky Wayne illustrates powerful, well-developed abdominal muscles. The dumbbell exercises (page 60), the calisthenics abdominal exercises (pages 42, 43) and the sit-up with barbell plate (page 106) produce good results. Ricky Wayne is the winner of "Mr. World" and "Mr. America" titles.

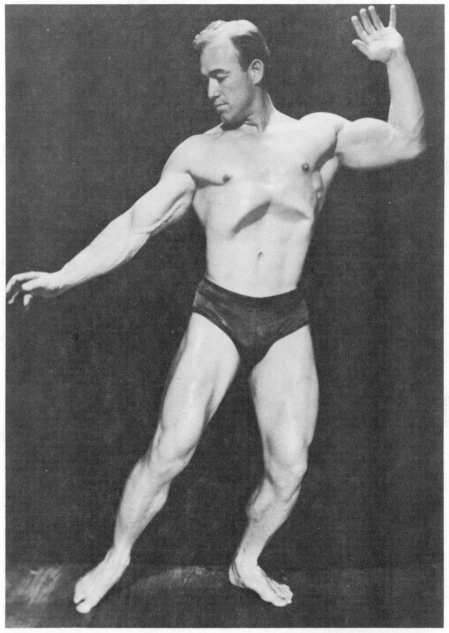

Fig. 53   Photo by Lon, New York City

An excellent example of well-defined, powerful thighs. The
knee-bend exercise with dumbbells (page 64) develops the thigh
muscles. For maximum development, do the deep knee-bend
exercise with barbells (pages 108, 109).

Pat Ryan, above, is well-known for his large, symmetrically
formed calves and thighs.

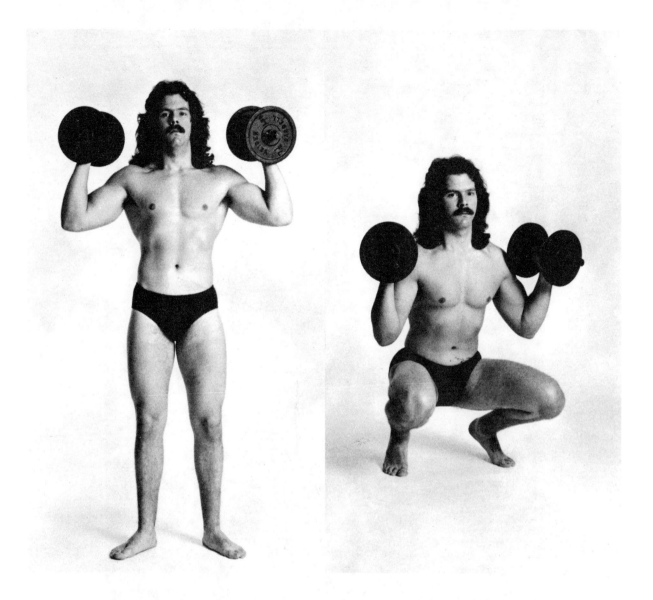

Fig. 54   Fig. 55

Lift 15 or 20 pound dumbbells to shoulders (*Fig. 54*). Take a deep breath, and lower yourself to squat position (*Fig. 55*). Then, exhale as you return to the upright position. Repeat 10 times. After several weeks, add one repetition each week, until you reach 15. For further development, add 5 pounds to each dumbbell and begin again with 10 repetitions.

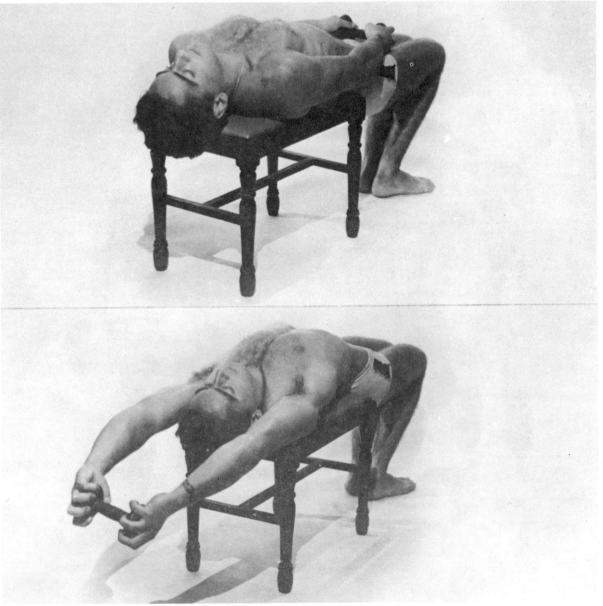

Fig. 56 (upper)   Fig. 57 (lower)

    Lie on a bench, or on the floor. Hold a 5 or 10 pound dumbbell at arm's length across your thighs (*Fig. 56*). Breathe in, and, with arms fully extended, raise the dumbbell overhead, and lower it to the back of your head (*Fig. 57*). Now, return weight overhead to original position and exhale. Begin with 10 repetitions. After several weeks, add one each week until you reach 15 repetitions.

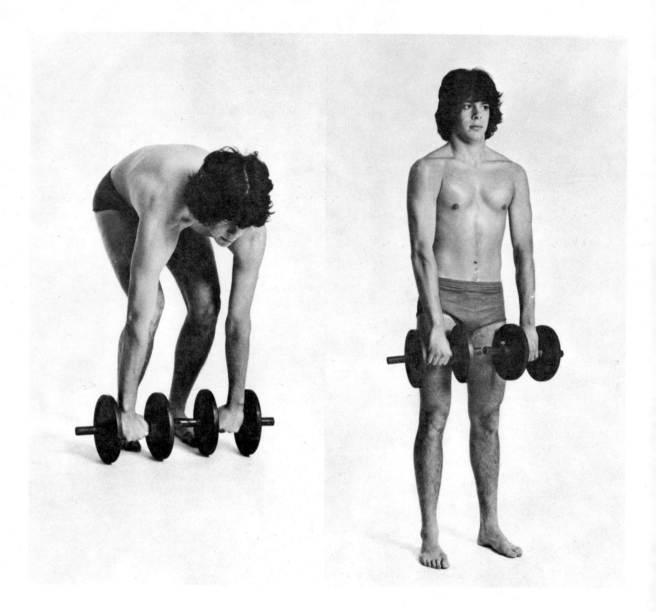

Fig. 58   Fig. 59

Place two 20 pound dumbbells on the floor before you. Bend your knees, and grasp the dumbbells, shoulder width apart (*Fig. 58*). Straighten up, holding the weights as shown in *Fig. 59*. Take a deep breath, and bend forward at the waist to a 90° angle (*Fig. 60*), and exhale. Breathe in deeply as you come to an erect position (*Fig. 61*). Repeat the exercise 10 times.

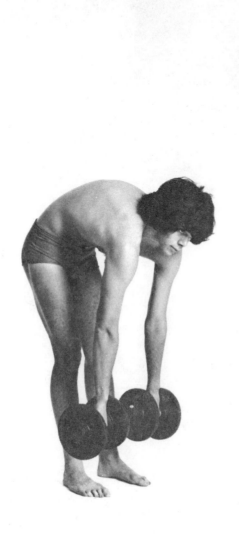
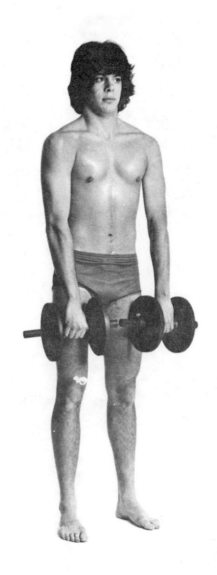

Fig. 60   Fig. 61

After several weeks, add one movement each week until you reach 15. For further development, add 5 pounds to each dumbbell and begin again with 10 repetitions.

A word of caution: when using heavy weights, bend the knees slightly to prevent possible strain to the lower back.

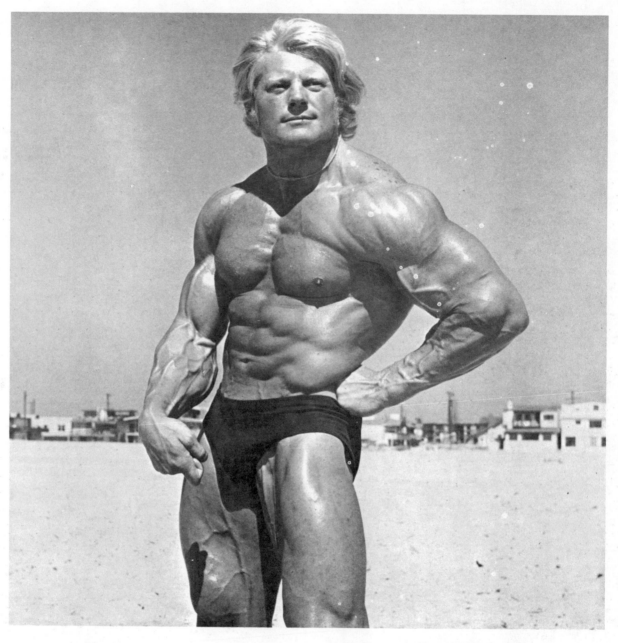

Fig. 62   Photo by Art Zeller, Santa Monica, Ca.

Dave Draper, above, shows a powerful set of trapezius muscles. The shoulder shrug (page 69) produces good results. For maximum development, see the shoulder shrug (page 116) and upright rowing (page 118). Dave Draper won the "Mr. Universe" and "Mr. America" titles.

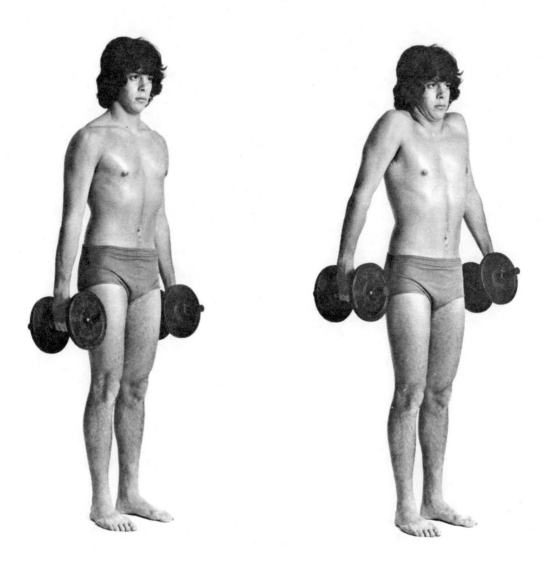

Fig. 63   Fig. 64

Hold two 15 or 20 pound dumbbells at your sides, with your arms fully extended down (*Fig. 63*). Raise your shoulders upward, in a shrug-like movement, and try to touch your ears (*Fig. 64*). Then, roll your shoulders all the way back and lower them to original position. Repeat 10 times. After several weeks, add one movement each week, until you reach 15. For further development, add 5 pounds and begin again with 10 repetitions.

69

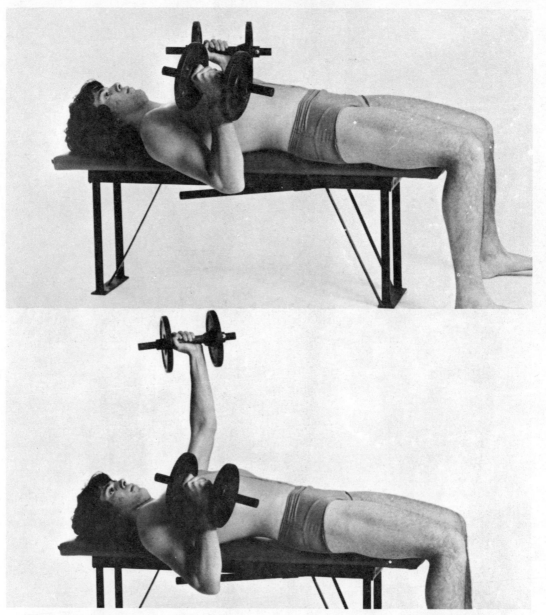

Fig. 65 (upper)   Fig. 66 (lower)

Place a 15 pound dumbbell on both sides of a low bench. Lie down, your back resting securely on bench, your head on one edge, and your buttocks just beyond the other. Lift dumbbells to your chest (*Fig. 65*). Press left dumbbell up (*Fig. 66*), inhaling as you go up. Exhale as you lower it and press the right dumbbell up. Repeat 10 times. After several weeks, add one movement a week, until you reach 15. For further development, add 5 pounds and begin again with 10 repetitions.

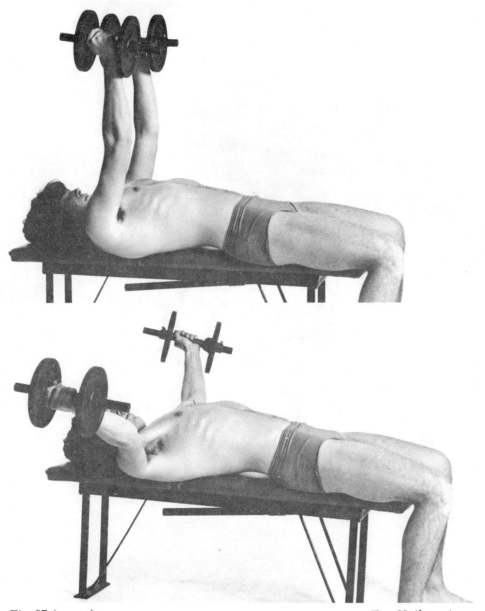

Fig. 67 (upper)   Fig. 68 (lower)

Assume same position as in the two-arm bench-press. Grasp two 5 or 10 pound dumbbells and bring them overhead, arms fully extended (*Fig. 67*). Breathe in as you lower the dumbbells to a horizontal position (*Fig. 68*), and exhale as you return weights to original position. Repeat 10 times. After several weeks, add an extra movement each week until you reach 15. For further development, add 5 pounds and begin again with 10 repetitions. This exercise may be done on a bench or floor.

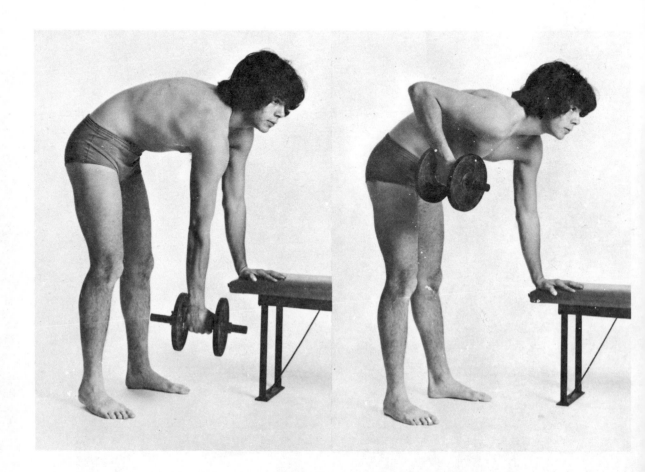

Fig. 69   Fig. 70

Grasp a 15 pound dumbbell in your right hand. Bend your body forward to a 90° angle. Rest left hand on a low stool or chair (*Fig. 69*). Inhale and raise right elbow as high as it will go (*Fig. 70*). Then, return to starting position (*Fig. 69*), and exhale. Reverse position and repeat with dumbbell in left hand. Repeat 10 times. After several weeks, add one movement each week, until you have reached 15. For further development, add 5 pounds and begin again with 10 repetitions.

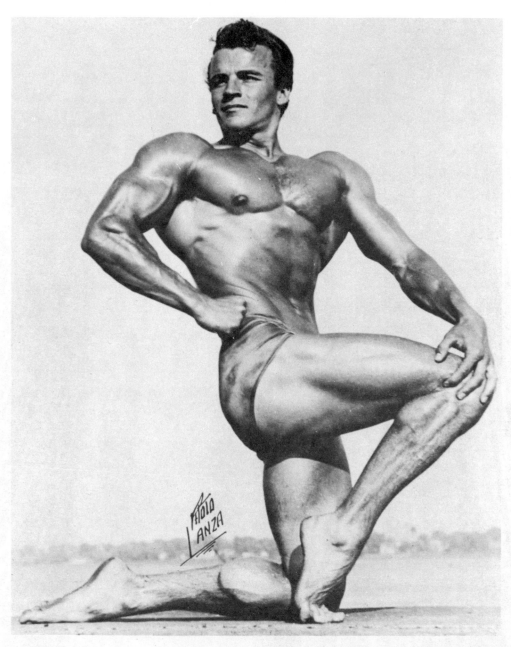

Fig. 71   Photo courtesy of Weider Publications, Jersey City, N. J.

Georges Boulanger, above, winner of a "Mr. Canada" title, shows the well-developed latissimus dorsi muscles. Pulleys (page 86) and the dumbbell rowing exercise (page 72), are effective exercises to develop these muscles. To attain peak development, do the chinning exercise (page 48).

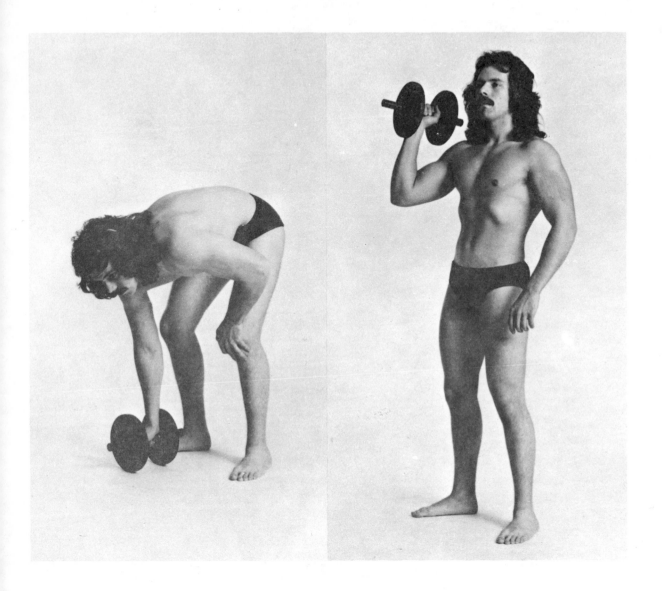

Fig. 72   Fig. 73

Place a 15 or 20 pound dumbbell between your feet. Bend forward and rest left hand on your left knee. Reach down and grasp the dumbbell with right hand (*Fig. 72*). Then, with a quick heave, lift it to shoulder level (*Fig. 73*). Now, press it overhead (*Fig. 74*), inhaling as you go up. In this position your arm is fully extended overhead, and in a straight vertical line with your shoulder and hip. Return the weight to your shoulder (*Fig. 75*), and exhale.

74

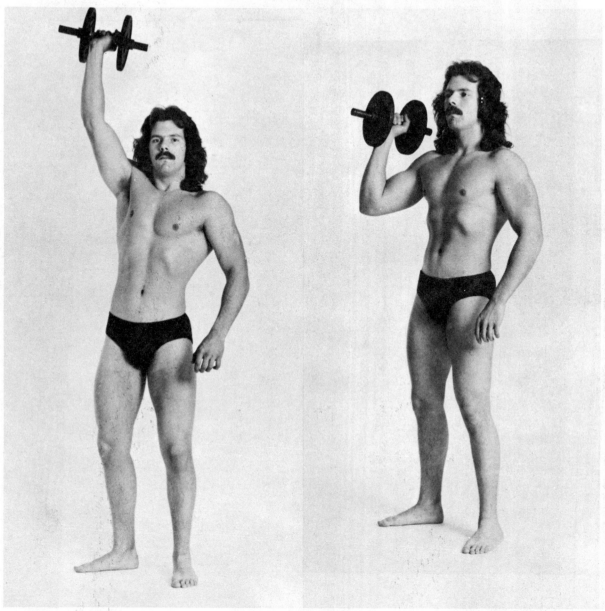

Fig. 74   Fig. 75

Change the dumbbell to left hand and repeat the full exercise. Perform this one-arm press 10 times, first with the right hand, and then with the left. After several weeks, add one movement a week until you reach 15. For further development, add 5 pounds and begin again with 10 repetitions.

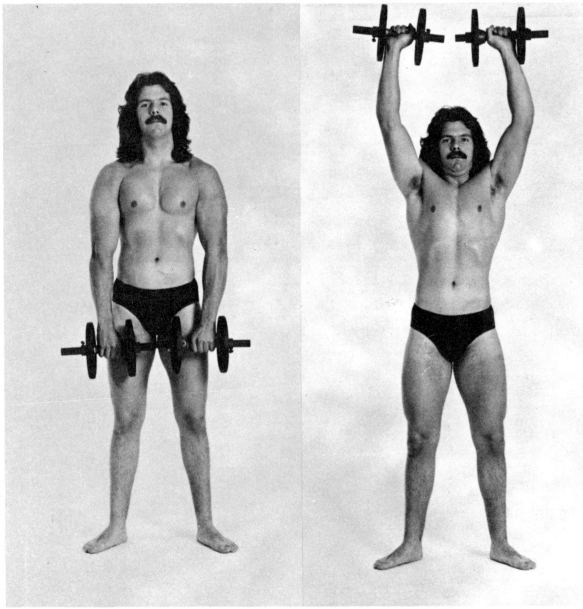

Fig. 76   Fig. 77

Hold 5 to 10 pound dumbbells in an overhand grip against the front of your thighs (*Fig. 76*). Raise your fully extended arms overhead, inhaling slowly, until they are straight up, in a vertical line with your body (*Fig. 77*). Exhale as you lower the dumbbells to your thighs. Repeat 10 times. Add one repetition each week, until you reach 15. Then, add 5 pounds and begin again with 10 repetitions.

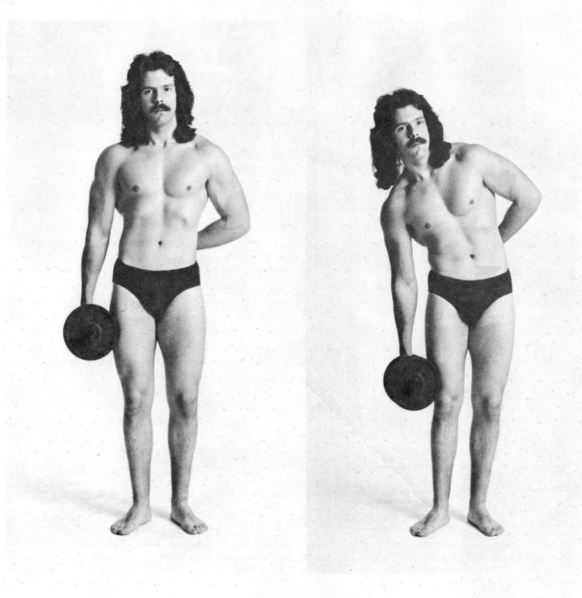

Fig. 78   Fig. 79

Grasp a 15 or 20 pound dumbbell in your right hand. Place your left hand behind your back and keep both feet together (*Fig. 78*). Now, bend sideways to the right as far as you can go (*Fig. 79*). From this position, swing over to the left side as far as possible. Alternate with your left hand. Repeat 10 times. After two weeks, add one movement each week until you reach 15. For further development, add 5 pounds and begin again with 10 repetitions.

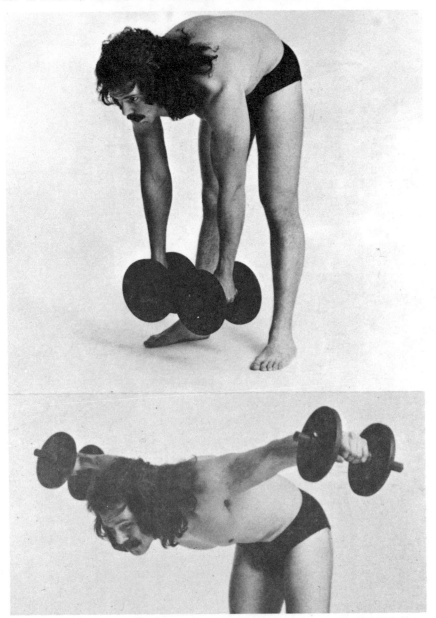

Fig. 80 (upper)   Fig. 81 (lower)

Grasp a 5 or 10 pound dumbbell in each hand. Bend your body forward to a 90° angle, arms hanging straight down (*Fig. 80*). Breathe in, and raise your arms horizontally, until the dumbbells are at shoulder level (*Fig. 81*). Exhale as you lower your arms to the starting position. Repeat each exercise 10 times. After several weeks, add an extra movement each week until you reach 15. For further development, add 5 pounds and begin again with 10 repetitions.

78

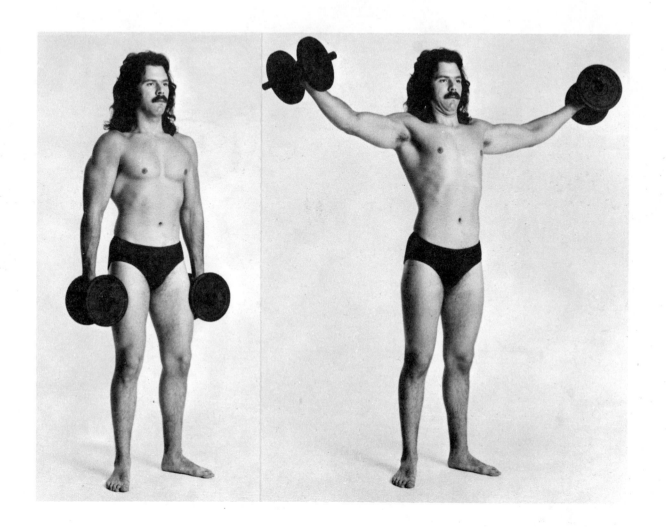

Fig. 82   Fig. 83

Grasp a 5 or 10 pound dumbbell in each hand and hold it alongside your body (*Fig. 82*). Slowly raise the dumbbells sideways (*Fig. 83*), until they are fully extended overhead. Inhale as you bring the weights up, and be sure not to bend your arms. Exhale slowly, as you lower arms to your side. Repeat 10 times. After several weeks, add one movement each week until you reach 15. For further development, add 5 pounds and begin again with 10 repetitions.

79

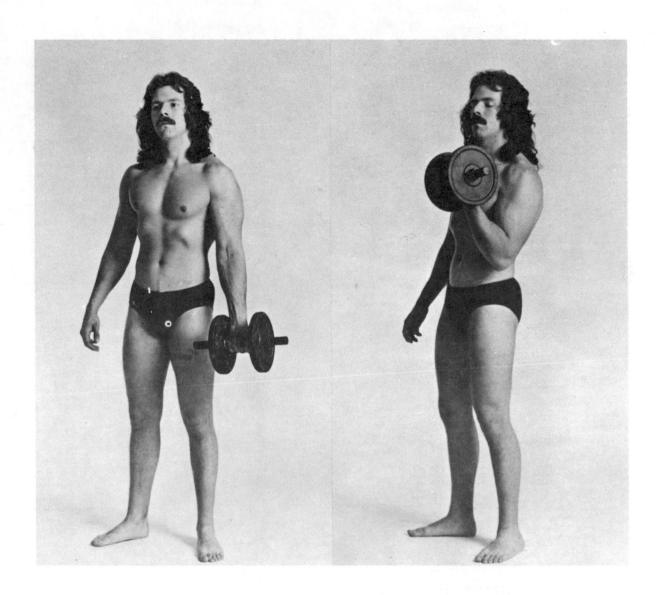

Fig. 84   Fig. 85

Stand erect and grasp a 10 or 15 pound dumbbell in your left hand with an underhand grip (*Fig. 84*). Bend your wrist toward you, curling the dumbbell slowly toward your shoulder (*Fig. 85*), inhaling as you go up. Return it to starting position at your side and exhale. Then, repeat with your right hand. Perform exercise 10 times. After several weeks, add one movement each week until you reach 15 repetitions. For further development, add 5 pounds and begin again with 10 repetitions.

80

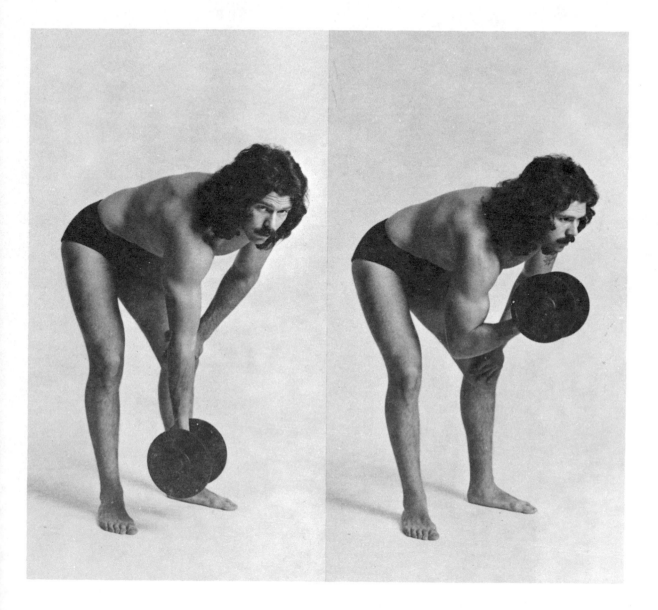

Fig. 86   Fig. 87

Bend your body to a 90° angle. Place your left hand on left knee. Grasp a 10 or 15 pound dumbbell with right hand (*Fig. 86*). Now, with your right arm held straight down, curl dumbbell toward your shoulder (*Fig. 87*), inhaling as you raise it, and exhaling as you lower it. Repeat exercise 10 times. After several weeks, add one movement a week until you reach 15 repetitions. For further development, add 5 pounds and begin again with 10 repetitions.

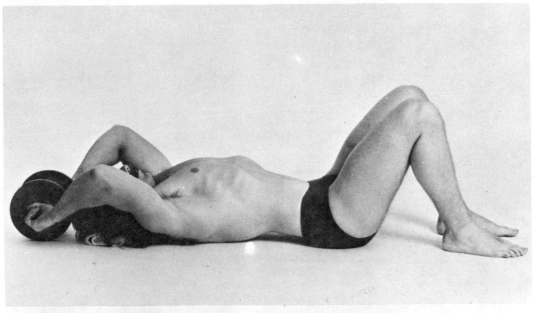

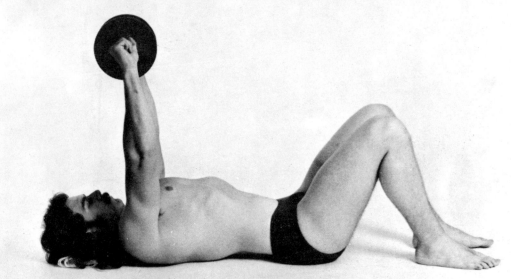

Fig. 88 (upper)   Fig. 89 (lower)

Lie on the floor, face up, with a towel or pad under your head and a 10 pound dumbbell directly behind your head. Raise your knees, keeping both feet flat on the floor. Reach back, and grasp the dumbbell with both hands (*Fig. 88*). Pull it over to your chest, and then press it overhead (*Fig. 89*). With the weight held in this vertical position, arch your back and neck to form

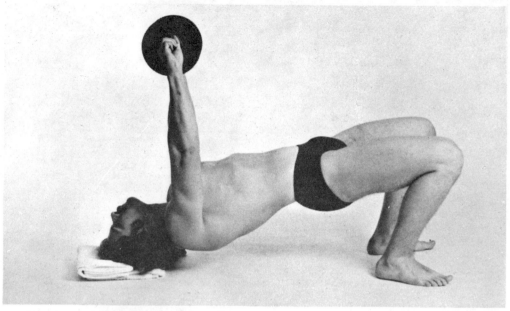

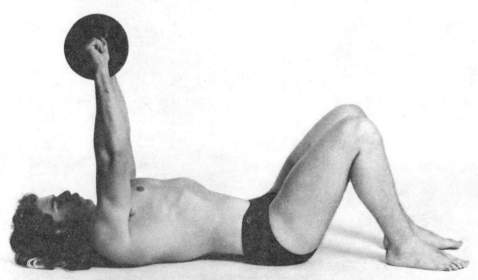

Fig. 90 (upper)   Fig. 91 (lower)

a bridge with your body (*Fig. 90*), inhaling as you arch. Then, lower your back and neck to the floor and exhale, keeping the weight overhead (*Fig. 91*). Begin with 10 repetitions. After a few weeks, add an extra movement each week until you reach 15. For further development, add 5 pounds and return to 10 repetitions.

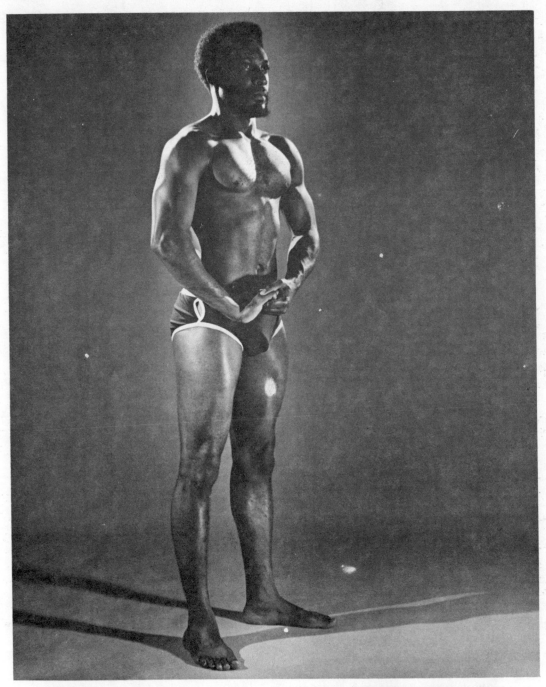

Fig. 92   Photographer Chas. Berman

John L. Brown developed this outstanding physique within five
short months training with barbells, dumbells and pulleys. John
gained twenty pounds of solid muscle. He put on 4″ on his chest, 2″
on his thighs and 1½″ on his arms. John expects to enter physique
competition in the near future.

Chapter 7

Pulley
Exercise Course

THE PULLEY course is an effective method for developing the upper muscles of the body. By combining the pulley course with the back, legs and abdominal exercises in the calisthenics chapter, you can increase the size and strength of all your muscles.

EXERCISE TO DEVELOP THE LATISSIMUS DORSI

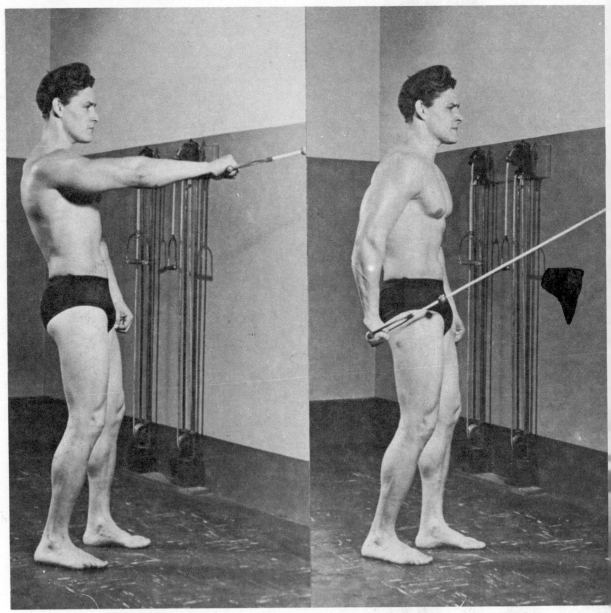

Fig. 93   Fig. 94

Attach a 10 pound weight to pulley. Face pulley, your feet 12 inches apart. Grasp pulley in overhand grip with right hand (*Fig. 93*), inhale and pull the weight down, bringing it back as far as it will go (*Fig. 94*). Return to starting position and exhale. Alternate by holding pulley in left hand. Repeat 10 times. After several weeks, add one movement each week until you reach 15. For further development, add a 5 pound weight to the pulley and return to 10 repetitions.

86

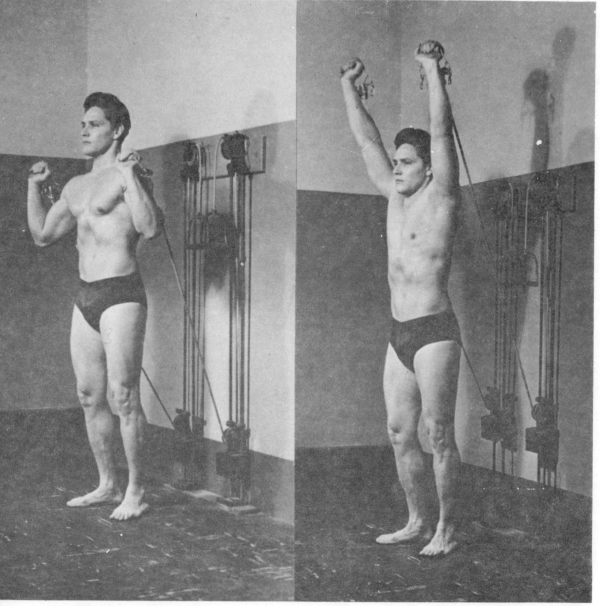

Fig. 95   Fig. 96

Attach a 15 pound weight to pulleys. Stand with your back to them. Grasp pulleys in overhand grip and raise them to your shoulders (*Fig. 95*). Then, inhale and press them overhead until both arms are fully extended upward (*Fig. 96*). Return to starting position (*Fig. 95*), and exhale. Repeat exercise 10 times. After several weeks, add one movement each week until you reach 15. For further development, add 5 pounds and return to 10 repetitions.

87

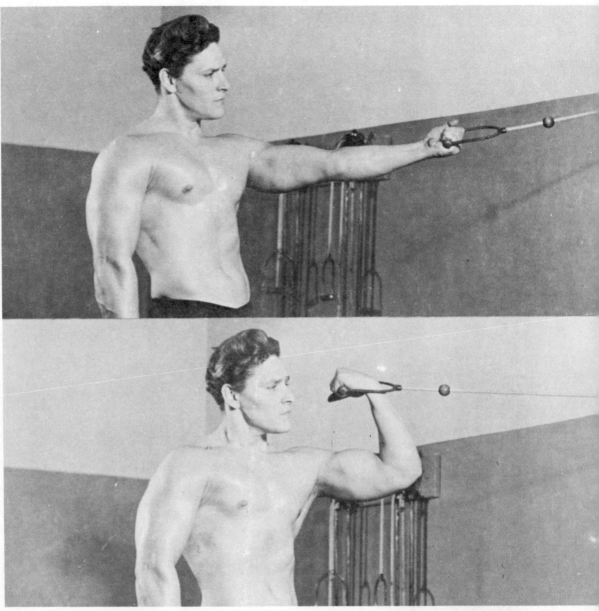

Fig. 97 (upper)   Fig. 98 (lower)

Attach a 10 or 15 pound weight to pulley. Grasp pulley in underhand grip with your left hand. Raise your arm, fully extended, to shoulder level (*Fig. 97*). Bend elbow and curl your wrist up to your left shoulder (*Fig. 98*). Return to starting position. Repeat exercise with right hand. Perform 10 times. After several weeks, add one curl each week until you reach 12. For further development, add a 2½ or 5 pound weight, and return to 10 repetitions.

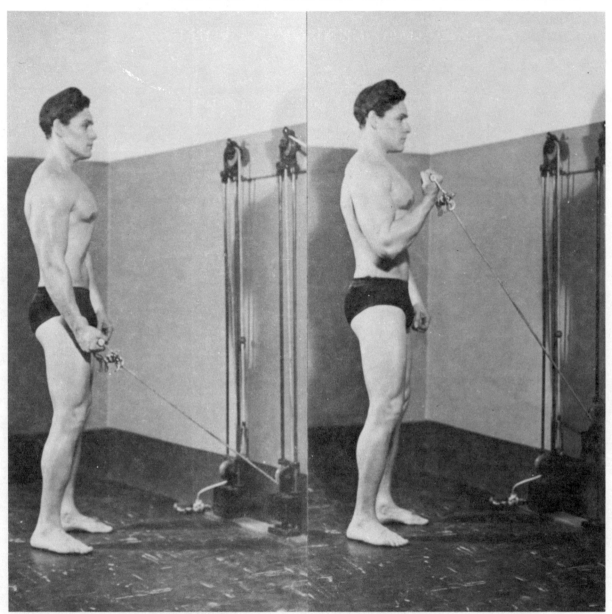

Fig. 99   Fig. 100

Attach a 10 or 15 pound weight to pulley. Grasp pulley in an underhand grip with right hand. Hold right arm close to your side (*Fig. 99*). Now, flex your arm, bringing the pulley up toward your right shoulder (*Fig. 100*). Then, return to starting position. Alternate by using your left hand. Repeat the exercise 10 times. After several weeks, add one curl each week until you reach 12. For further development, add 2½ to 5 pound weights and return to 10 repetitions.

89

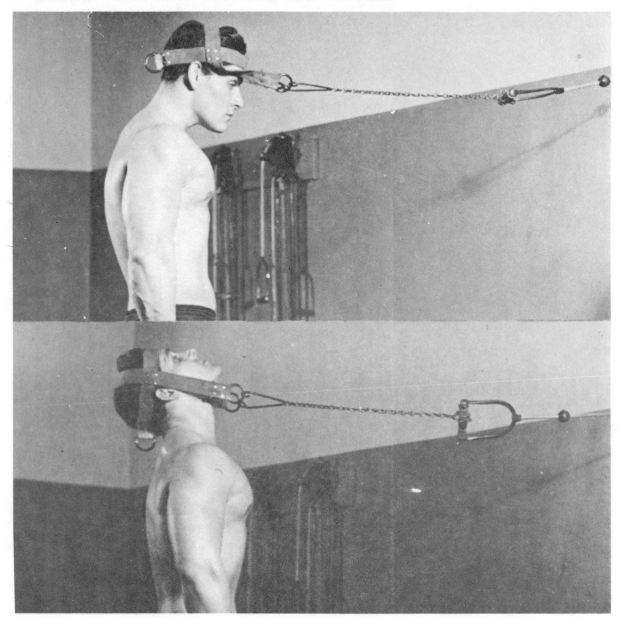

Fig. 101 (upper)   Fig. 102 (lower)

This exercise requires a headgear, one end of which fits on to your head; the other end is attached to the pulley.

Attach a 5 or 10 pound weight to pulley. Facing the pulley, put on headgear, your chin resting on your chest. Raise your head (*Fig. 101*), and bring it back as far as you can (*Fig. 102*). Then, return to starting position.

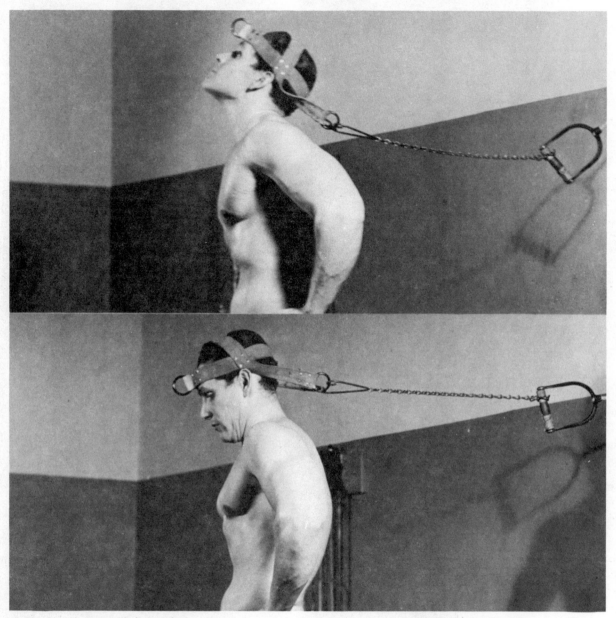

Fig. 103 (upper)   Fig. 104 (lower)

Put headgear on. Stand with your back to pulley, your head held as far back as possible (*Fig. 103*). Bring your head forward (*Fig. 104*) until your chin touches your chest. Now, return to starting position.

Repeat both exercises 10 times. After several weeks, add one movement each week until you reach 15. For further development, add 2½ or 5 pound weights and return to 10 repetitions.

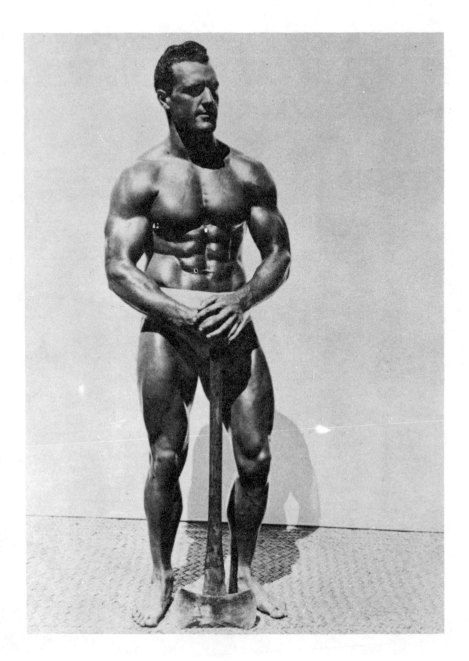

Fig. 105   Photo courtesy of Weider Publications, Jersey City, N. J.

Clarence "Clancy" Ross, above, shows well-developed front and side deltoid muscles. The two-arm press with barbells (page 103), and the front lateral raise with barbells (page 122) are for developing the front deltoids. For side deltoids, do the two-arm press behind neck (page 119) and the side lateral raise with dumbbells (page 79).

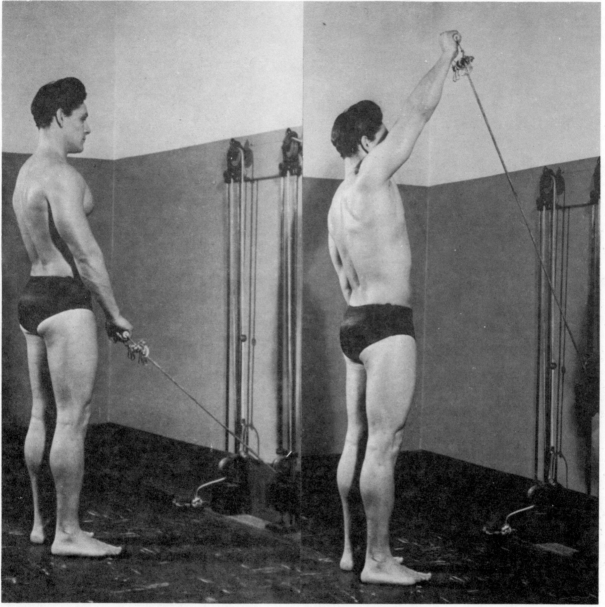

Fig. 106   Fig. 107

Attach a 5 pound weight to floor pulley. Face the pulley, grasping it in an overhand grip with your right hand (*Fig. 106*). With your arm fully extended, inhale and bring the pulley overhead (*Fig. 107*). Return to starting position and exhale. Change to your left arm and repeat. Perform the exercise 10 times. After several weeks, add one movement each week, until you reach 15. For further development, add 2½ pound weights and return to 10 repetitions.

93

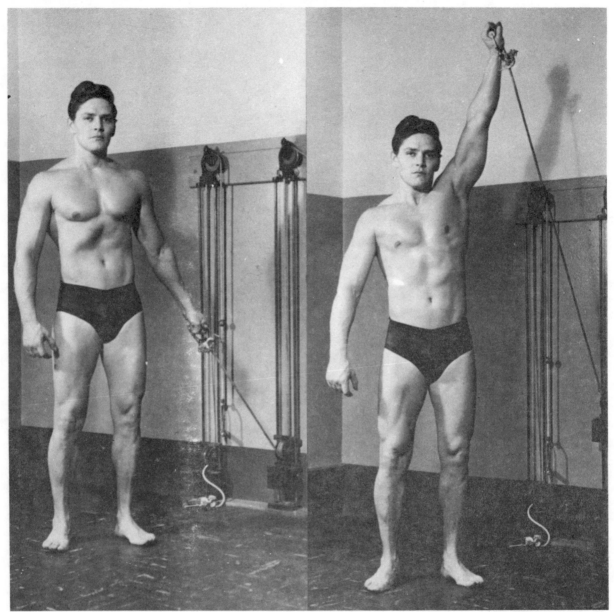

Fig. 108   Fig. 109

Attach a 5 pound weight to pulley. Grasp pulley in an over-hand grip with left hand, turning the left side of your body into line with it (*Fig. 108*). With your arm fully extended, inhale and raise pulley overhead (*Fig. 109*). Return to starting position and exhale. Repeat with right hand. Perform 10 times with each hand. After several weeks, add one movement each week until you reach 15. For further development, add a 2½ pound weight and return to 10 repetitions.

94

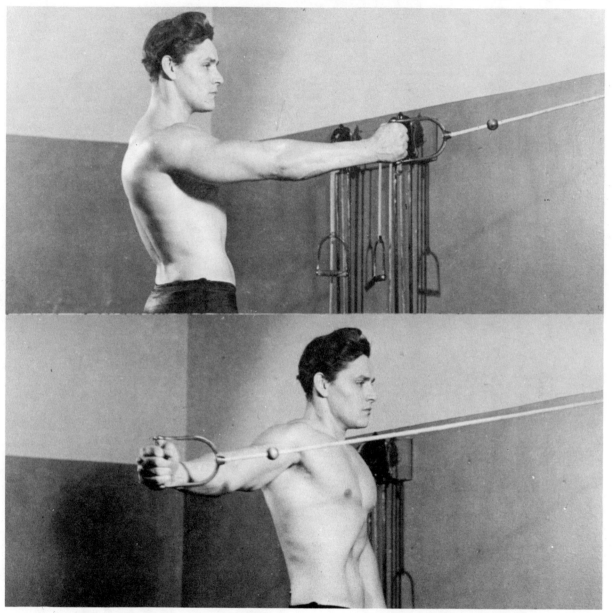

Fig. 110 (upper)   Fig. 111 (lower)

Attach a 5 pound weight to pulley. Face pulley with your feet 12 inches apart. Grasp it in an overhand grip with your right hand, at shoulder level (*Fig. 110*). With your arm held straight out, inhale, and draw the pulley sideways as far back as you can go (*Fig. 111*). Return to original position and exhale. Repeat 10 times with each hand. After several weeks, add one movement a week, until you reach 15. For further development, add 2½ or 5 pounds, and return to 10 repetitions.

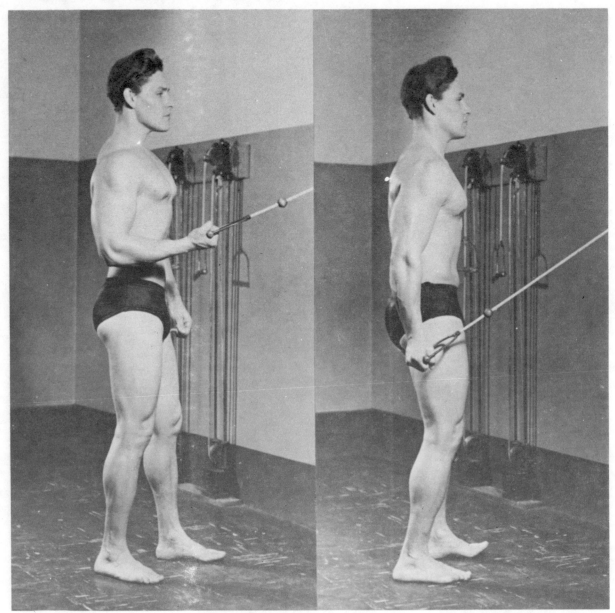

Fig. 112   Fig. 113

Attach a 5 to 10 pound weight to wall pulley. Grasp the pulley in an underhand grip with right hand, your forearms bent to a 90° angle (*Fig. 112*). Then, draw pulley down as far as it will go (*Fig. 113*). Now, return to the starting position. Repeat with the left hand. Perform 10 repetitions. After several weeks, add one movement each week until you reach 15. For further development, add a 2½ or 5 pound weight and return to 10 repetitions.

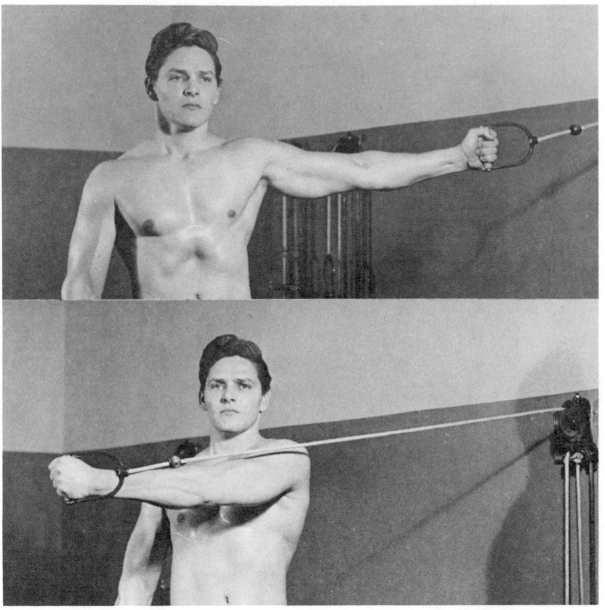

Fig. 114 (upper)   Fig. 115 (lower)

Attach a 5 pound weight to floor pulley. Grasp pulley in overhand grip with left hand, and raise your arm to shoulder level. Assume the position in *Fig. 114*. With arm held straight out, bring the pulley across your chest (*Fig. 115*); then return to starting position (*Fig. 114*). Repeat with the right hand. Perform 10 times with each hand. After several weeks, add one movement each week until you reach 15. For further development, add 2½ pounds, and return to 10 repetitions.

97

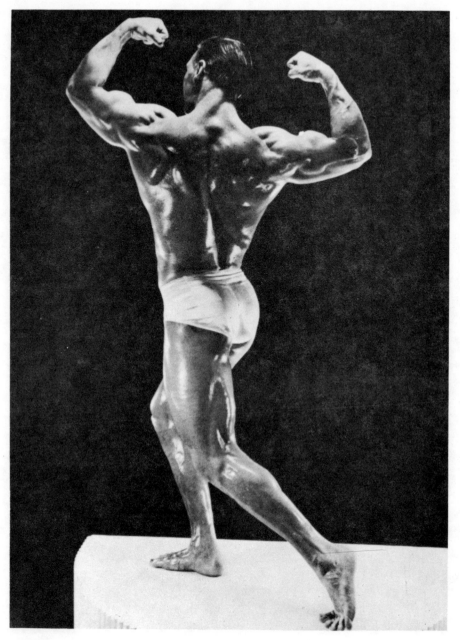

Fig. 116   Photo courtesy of Weider Publications, Jersey City, N. J.

Floyd Page, above, shows his powerful, well-defined erector spinal muscles. The advanced back exercise in the Calisthenics course (pages 38, 39), and the dead weight lift with barbells (pages 114, 115), develop the spinal erectae muscles.

Chapter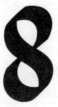

Barbell
Exercise Course

BARBELL EXERCISES are, by far, the quickest and the most effective way to attain all-around muscular development.

Louis Rodriguez, the model for the barbell course, is 18 years of age, and has already attained a magnificently proportioned and well-developed physique.

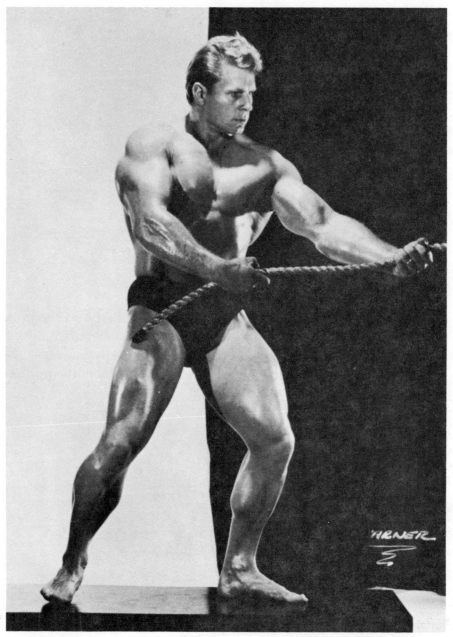

Fig. 117   Photo courtesy of Weider Publications, Jersey City, N. J.

Jack Delinger, above, is an outstanding example of what can be achieved through barbell exercises. He is well-known for his truly Herculean physique. Among his many awards are "Mr. America," "Mr. Western America," and "Mr. Northern California."

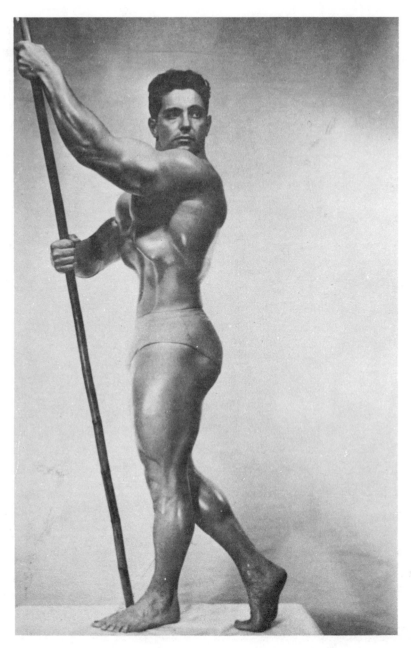

Fig. 118   Photo by Lon, New York City

This photo of Abe Goldberg, renown for his magnificently proportioned physique, illustrates a well-developed rib-box. The two-arm pullover with dumbbells (page 65) will develop the rib-box. Abe Goldberg operates his own gym in New York City.

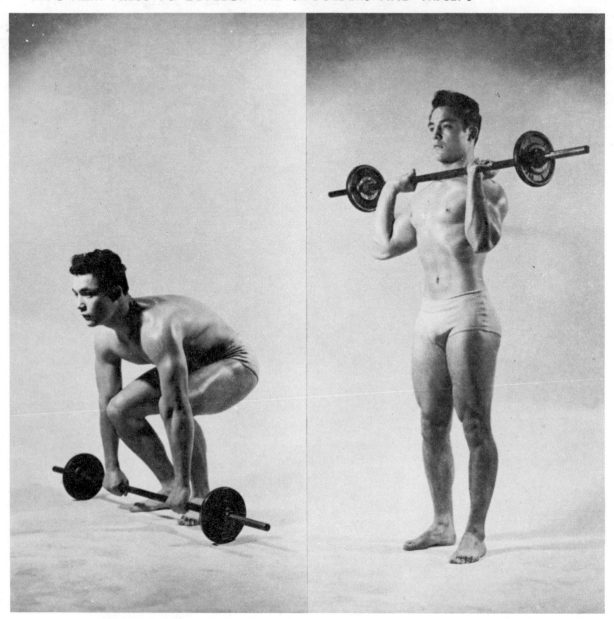

Fig. 119   Fig. 120

Place a 30 or 40 pound barbell before you, your feet 12 inches apart. Bend down and grasp barbell, your hands about shoulder width apart (*Fig. 119*). *Your knees must be bent.* Take a deep breath, and lift the weight to your chest with a quick heave (*Fig. 120*); then exhale. You must coordinate the arms, legs and back in *one continuous movement* when you lift the weight to your chest. From this position, take a deep breath and

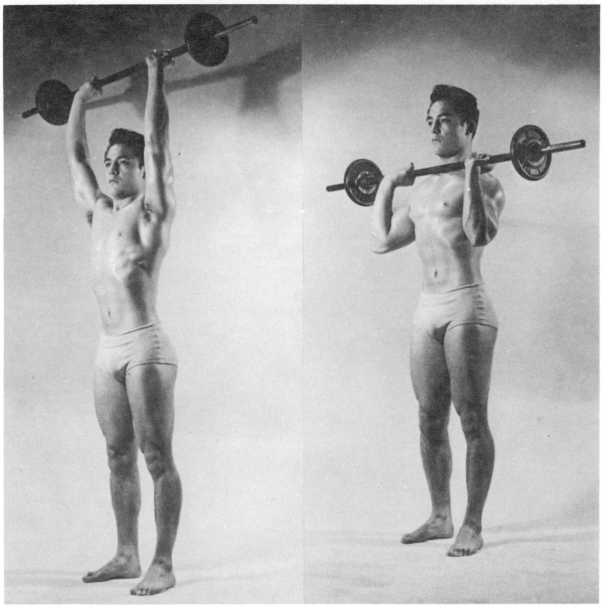

Fig. 121   Fig. 122

press the weight straight up overhead (*Fig. 121*). Then, return it to the chest at shoulder level (*Fig. 122*), and exhale. You need not return weight to floor to continue exercise. Raise and lower it from shoulder level. Repeat 10 times. After several weeks, increase repetitions by one each week until you reach 15. For further development, add 5 pounds and begin again with 10 repetitions. Try different weights in the beginning to find one you can easily press up 10 times.

103

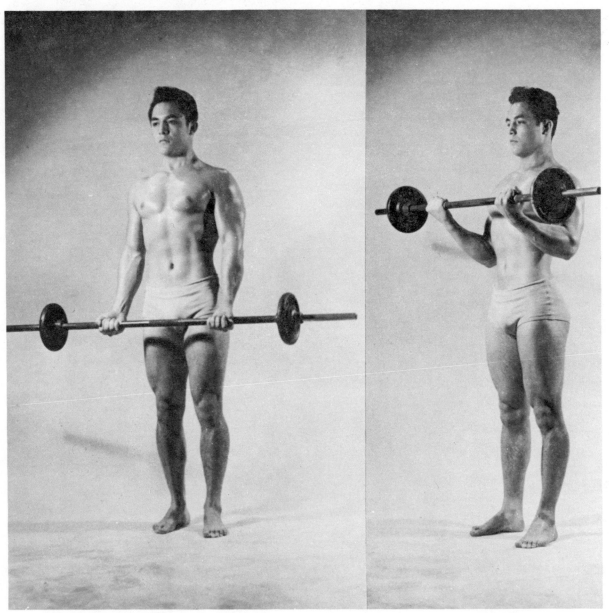

Fig. 123   Fig. 124

Grasp a 15 or 25 pound barbell with both hands, shoulder width apart, using the underhand grip (*Fig. 123*). Bend your wrists toward you and curl the weight toward your shoulder (*Fig. 124*), inhaling as you go up. Return to the starting position (*Fig. 123*), and exhale. Repeat 10 times. After several weeks, add one repetition each week until you reach a total of 15. Then, add 5 pounds to the weight, and begin again with 10 repetitions.

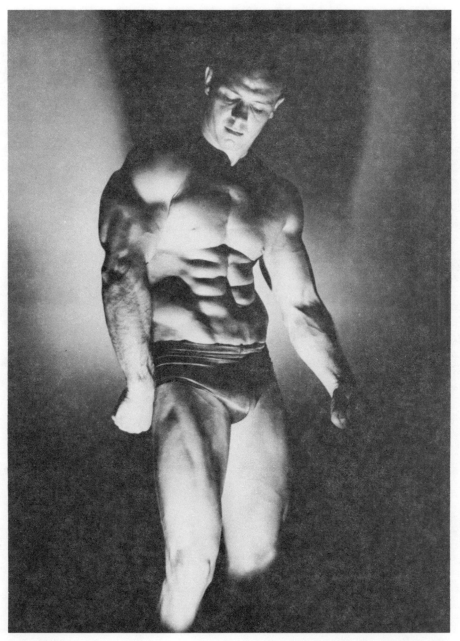

Fig. 125   Photo by Bruce of Los Angeles

This photo of Irvin Koszewski illustrates well-knit, power-ful upper and lower abdominal muscles. Sit-ups with dumb-bells (pages 60, 61) is the best way to develop these muscles. Sit-ups with barbell plate (page 106), and abdominal calis-thenic exercises (pages 42, 43) will produce good results where no dumbbells are available. Mr. Koszewski has won the "best abdominal" awards at several "Mr. America" contests, in addi-tion to the "Mr. California" title.

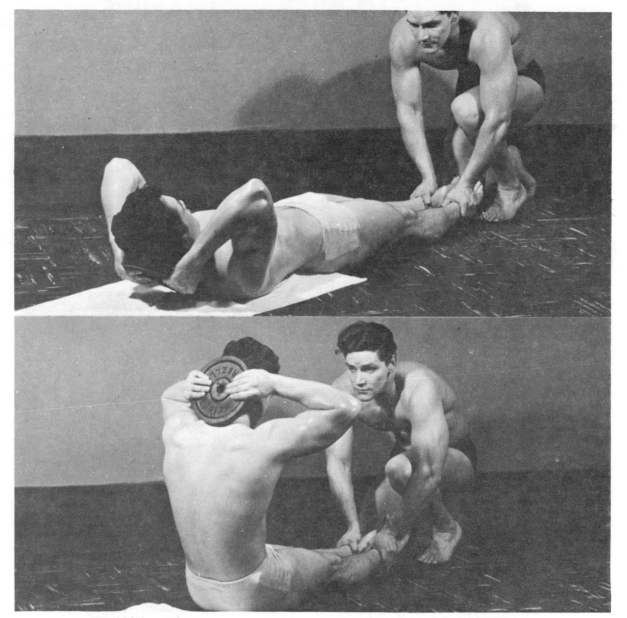

Fig. 126 (upper)   Fig. 127 (lower)

You are ready to sit up with weights after two months of calisthenic abdominal exercises. Begin with 5 pound plate. Lie flat on your back, holding the plate behind your head (*Fig. 126*). Place your feet below a heavy, stationary object, or, have someone hold them in place. Take a deep breath, and sit up, exhaling as you go (*Fig. 127*). Now, slowly lower your back to the floor. Repeat 10 times. After several weeks, add one repetition each week until you reach 15.

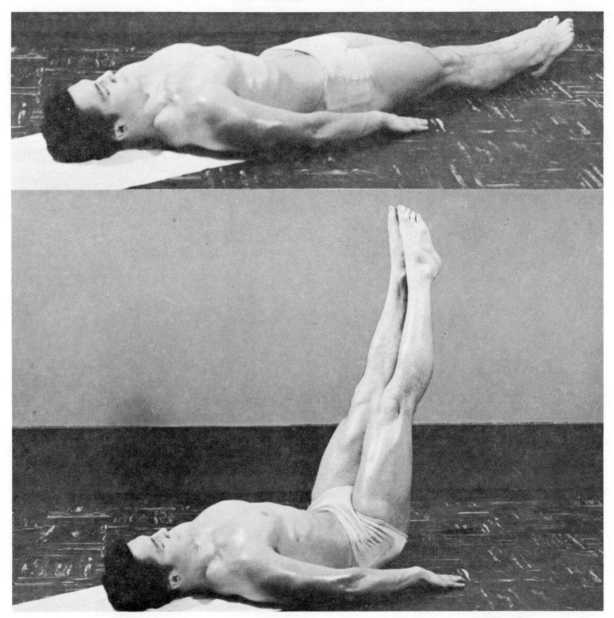

Fig. 128 (upper)   Fig. 129 (lower)

To exercise the lower abdominals, assume position in *Fig. 128*, hands next to sides, palms touching the floor. Take a deep breath, and raise both feet to a 90° angle (*Fig. 129*). Then, lower legs to floor, and exhale. Keep legs straight throughout the exercise. Repeat 5 times. After several weeks, add one repetition each week, until you reach 25.

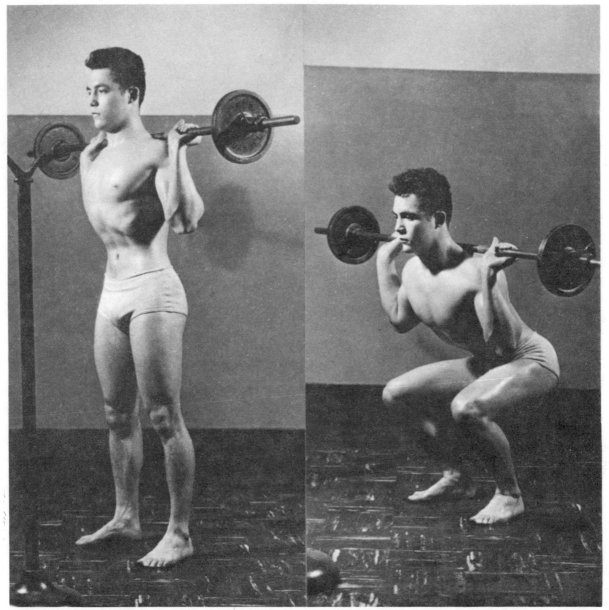

Fig. 130   Fig. 131

Place a 30 or 40 pound barbell across the upper back and shoulders, with your feet about twelve inches apart (*Fig. 130*). Take a deep breath, and lower your body, until your thighs are parallel to the floor (*Fig. 131*). Exhale as you return to starting position (*Fig. 132*). Repeat 10 times. After several weeks, add one movement each week until you reach 15.

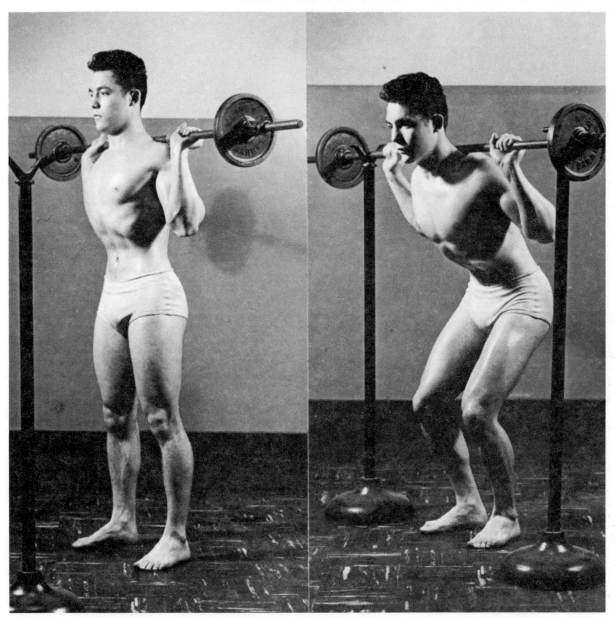

Fig. 132   Fig. 133

For further development, add 10 pounds and return to 10 repetitions. As you increase the weights for the knee-bend, it may be advisable to use knee-bend stands (*Fig. 133*). This makes it easier to lift heavy weights off the stands and put them back on again at the completion of the exercise, without straining other parts of the body.

109

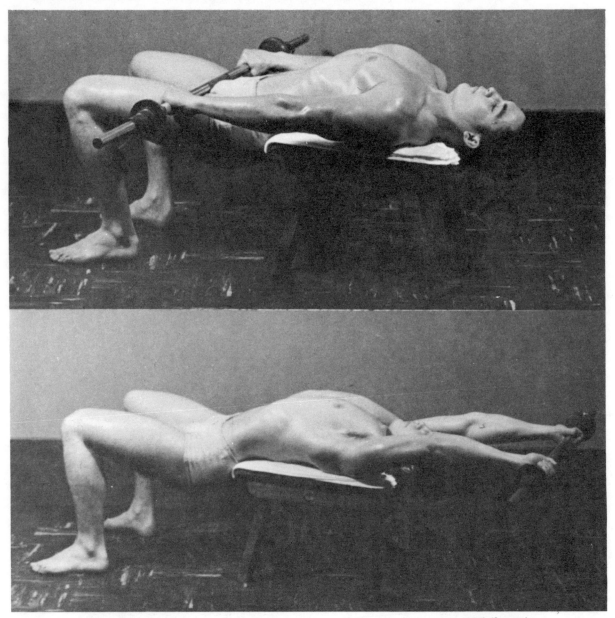

Fig. 134 (upper)   Fig. 135 (lower)

Lie on a bench. Place a 10 or 20 pound bar across your thighs at arms length (*Fig. 134*). Breathe in as you lift weight to the back of your head with your arms fully extended (*Fig. 135*). Return the bar overhead to original position (*Fig. 134*), and exhale. Begin with 10 repetitions. After several weeks, increase by one each week until you reach 15. For further development, add 5 pounds, and return to 10 repetitions. This exercise can also be done lying on the floor.

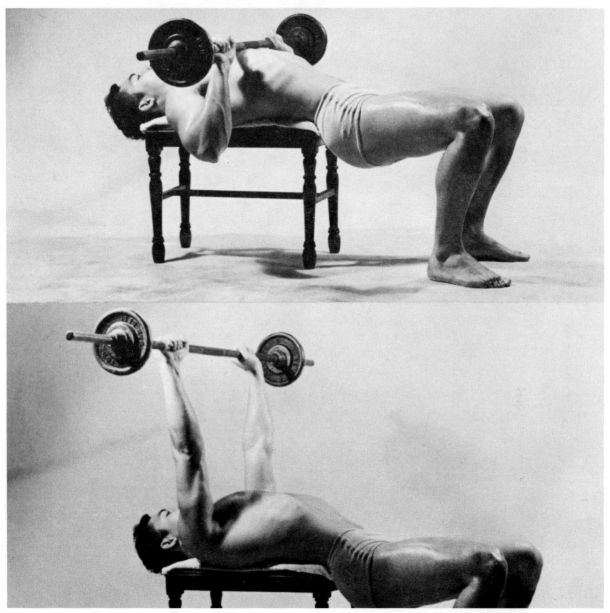

Fig. 136 (upper)   Fig. 137 (lower)

Lie flat on bench; place a 30 or 40 pound barbell across your chest, holding it shoulder width apart, in an overhand grip (*Fig. 136*). Press weight overhead at arms length (*Fig. 137*), inhaling as you raise it. Then, exhale as you return weight to starting position. Repeat 10 times. After several weeks, add one movement each week until you reach 15. For further development add 5 pounds to the barbell, and return to 10 repetitions. Exercise can also be done lying on the floor.

111

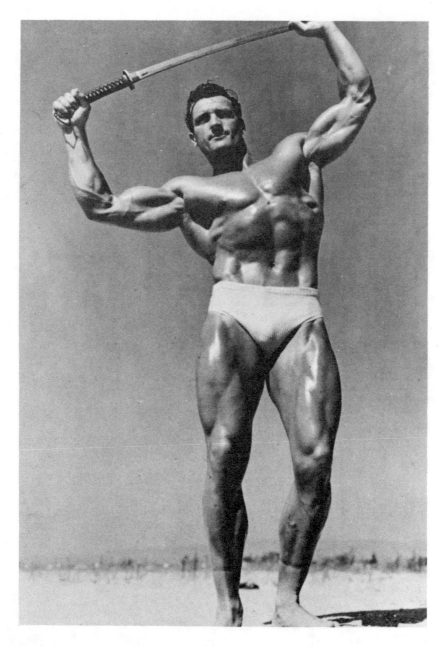

Fig. 138   Photo courtesy of Weider Publications, Jersey City, N. J.

This photo of Clarence "Clancy" Ross illustrates well-developed and well-defined external oblique muscles. The side exercise on page 113 is the most effective one for achieving maximum results. Mr. Ross has won just about every contest he entered.

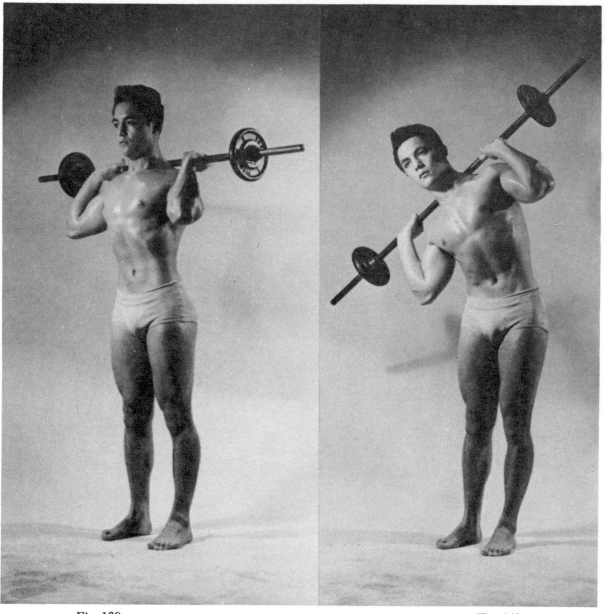

Fig. 139   Fig. 140

Stand erect, feet about 12 inches apart, with a 20 pound barbell across the back of your shoulders (*Fig. 139*). Be sure that the barbell collars are securely fastened. Bend sideways to the right as far as you can go (*Fig. 140*), then bend all the way to the left, and return to original position (*Fig. 139*). After several weeks, add one movement a week until you reach 15. Then add 5 pounds and begin again with 10 repetitions.

113

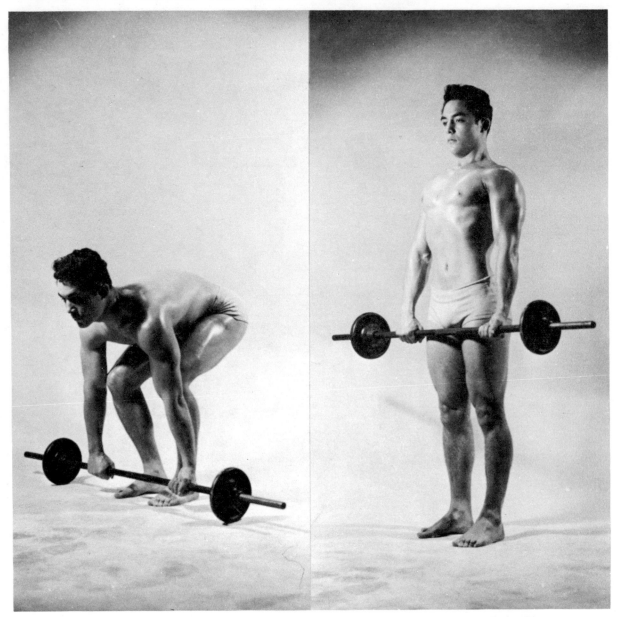

Fig. 141   Fig. 142

Place your feet 12 inches apart. Bend your knees and grasp a 30 to 40 pound weight, shoulder width apart, using the left hand in an underhand grip, and the right hand in an overhand grip (*Fig. 141*). Now, straighten up as in *Fig. 142*. Take a deep breath and bend forward until your body forms a 90° angle (*Fig. 143*), then exhale. This movement will lower the weight to a position halfway between your knees and ankles. Inhale as you

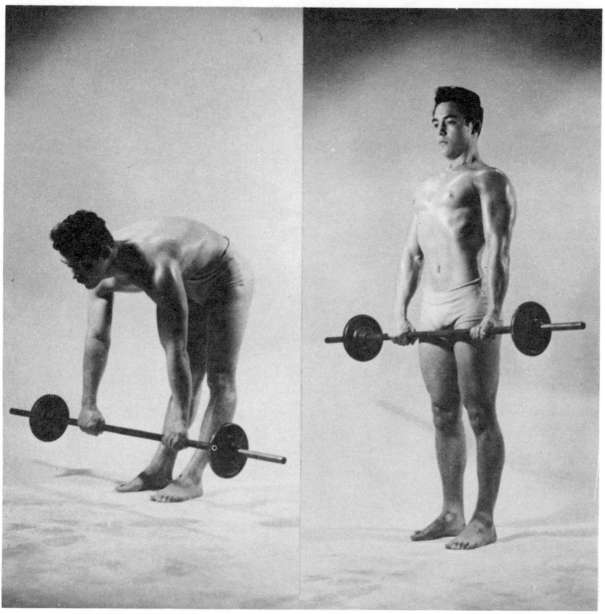

Fig. 143   Fig. 144

return to erect position (*Fig. 144*). Repeat 10 times. Add one
movement each week until you reach 15. For further development, increase the weight by 5 or 10 pounds and return to 10
repetitions. It is not necessary to lower weight beyond a position halfway between your knees and ankles. A word of caution:
When you use heavy weights, bend your knees as you lift. This
takes strain off lower back.

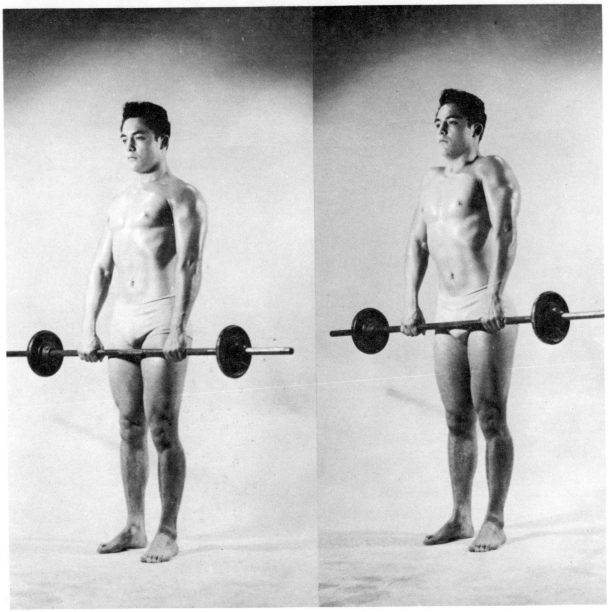

Fig. 145   Fig. 146

Hold a 30 or 40 pound barbell against your thighs, shoulder width apart, arms fully extended (*Fig. 145*). Raise shoulders, and bring them as close to your ears as you can (*Fig. 146*), inhaling as you go up. Now, bring shoulders as far back as they will go; then lower shoulders and arms to original position (*Fig. 145*), and exhale. Repeat 10 times. After several weeks, add one movement each week until you reach 15. For further development, add 5 pounds and begin with 10 repetitions.

116

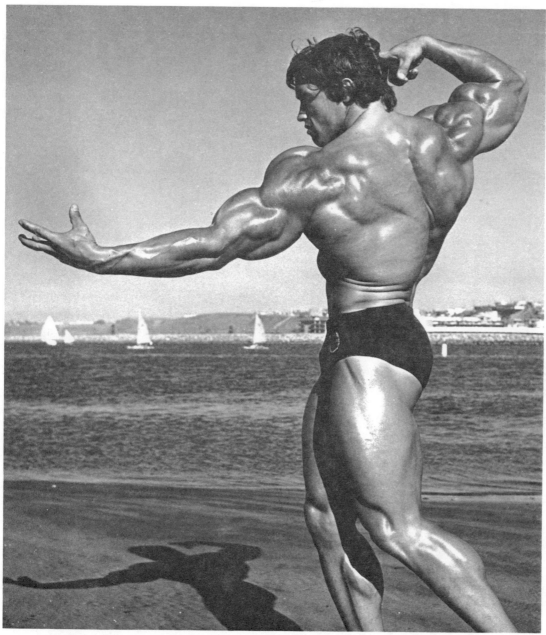

Fig. 147   Photo by Art Zeller, Santa Monica, Ca.

Arnold Schwarzenegger, above, shows well-developed triceps. The bench press (page 111), the two-arm press (pages 102, 103) and the two-arm press behind neck (page 119) are effective tricep exercises. Arnold Schwarzenegger won the "Mr. Olympia," "Mr. Universe" and "Mr. World" titles.

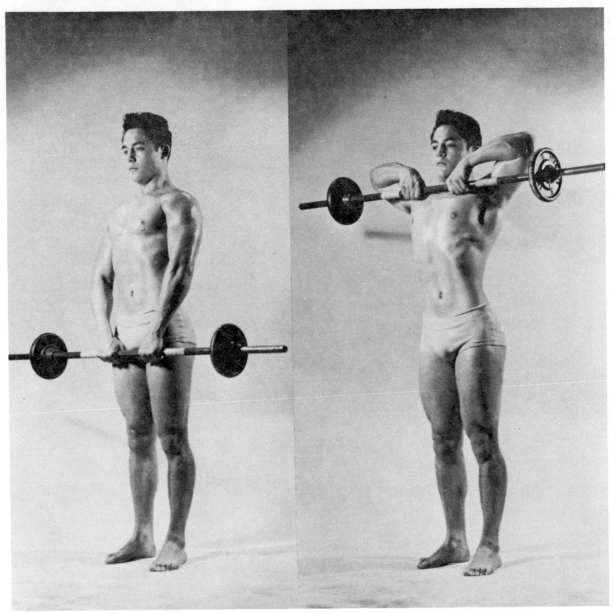

Fig. 148   Fig. 149

Grasp a 20 pound barbell in an overhand grip with both hands at the center of the bar, 4 inches apart (*Fig. 148*). Hold weight against the thighs, arms fully extended down. From this position, inhale and pull weight toward the neck (*Fig. 149*). Then, exhale as you lower it to original position (*Fig. 148*). Repeat 10 times. After several weeks, add one movement each week until you reach 15. For further development, add 5 pounds and begin with 10 repetitions.

118

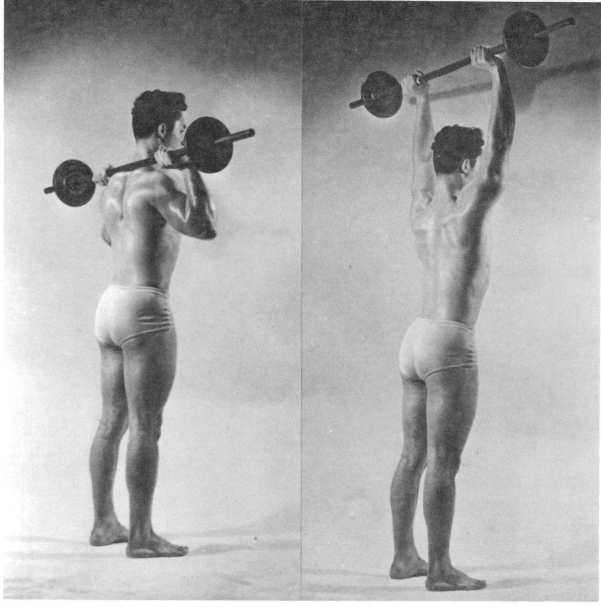

Fig. 150   Fig. 151

Stand erect, feet about 12 inches apart. Place a 15 to 25 pound barbell across the back of your shoulders (*Fig. 150*). Take a deep breath and press the weight overhead (*Fig. 151*). Then, slowly lower the weight to the back of the neck and exhale (*Fig. 150*). Repeat the exercise 10 times. Add one movement each week until you reach a total of 15. For further development, add 5 pounds and return to 10 repetitions.

119

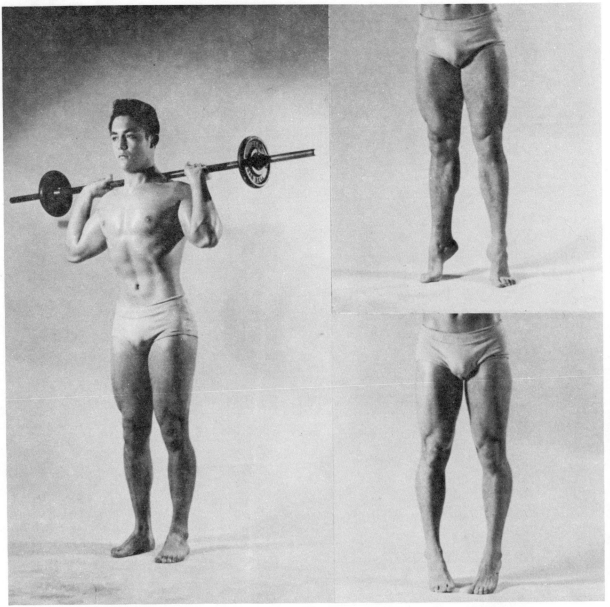

Fig. 152   Fig. 153 (upper)   Fig. 154 (lower)

Lift a 30 or 40 pound barbell overhead, and place it across the back of your shoulders, feet 12 inches apart, toes parallel to each other (*Fig. 152*). Then, rise on toes as high as you can go, keeping your body erect. Now, lower your heels to floor. Repeat exercise with toes pointing out (*Fig. 153*) and in (*Fig. 154*). Perform 10 times. After several weeks, add one movement each week until you reach 15. For further development, add 5 pounds and return to 10 repetitions.

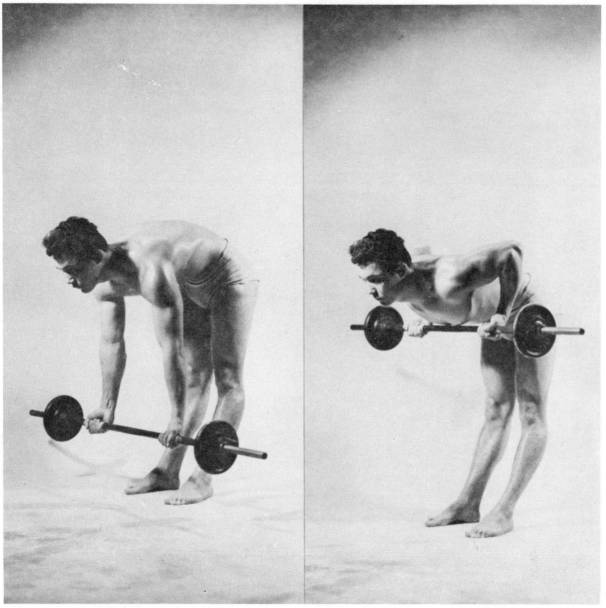

Fig. 155   Fig. 156

Grasp a 20 to 30 pound barbell in an underhand grip, shoulder width apart. Stand erect, with your feet about 12 inches apart. Now, bend your body forward, to a 90° angle (*Fig. 155*). Inhale and pull the weight as close to your chest as it will go (*Fig. 156*). Then, return weight to starting position (*Fig. 155*), and exhale. Repeat 10 times. After several weeks, add one movement each week until you reach a total of 15. For further development, add 5 pounds and return to 10 repetitions.

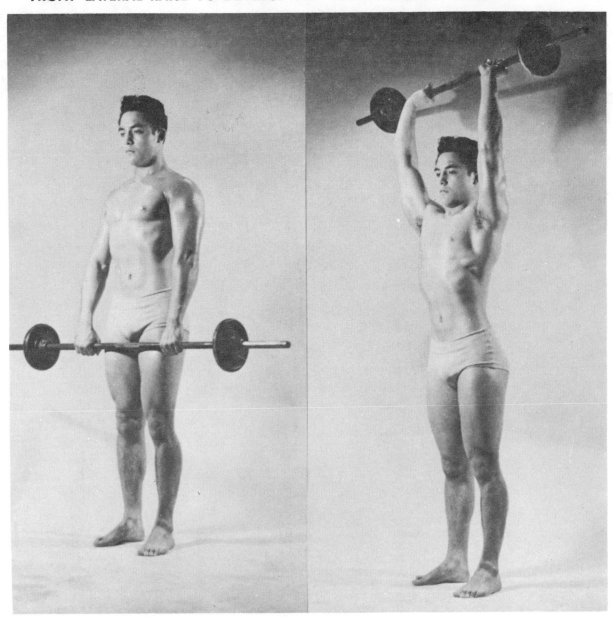

Fig. 157   Fig. 158

Hold a 15 pound barbell, arms fully extended downward, in an overhand grip, shoulder width apart, resting against your thighs (*Fig. 157*). Keep your arms straight and slowly raise the barbell upward in front of you until it reaches a position directly overhead (*Fig. 158*). Inhale as you go up, and exhale as you lower the weight. Repeat 10 times. After several weeks, add one movement each week until you reach 15. For further development, add 5 pounds and return to 10 repetitions.

122

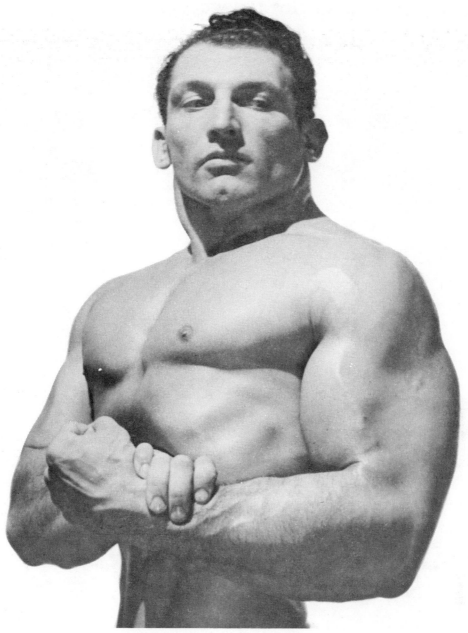

Fig. 159   Photo by Spartan of Hollywood

Everett Sinderoff, above, displays a sturdy, well-muscled
neck. Neck muscles can best be developed by the wrestler's
bridge exercise with barbells (pages 124, 125). Calisthenic neck
exercise (pages 40, 41), and wrestler's bridge with dumbbells
(pages 82, 83), are also effective for building the neck muscles.

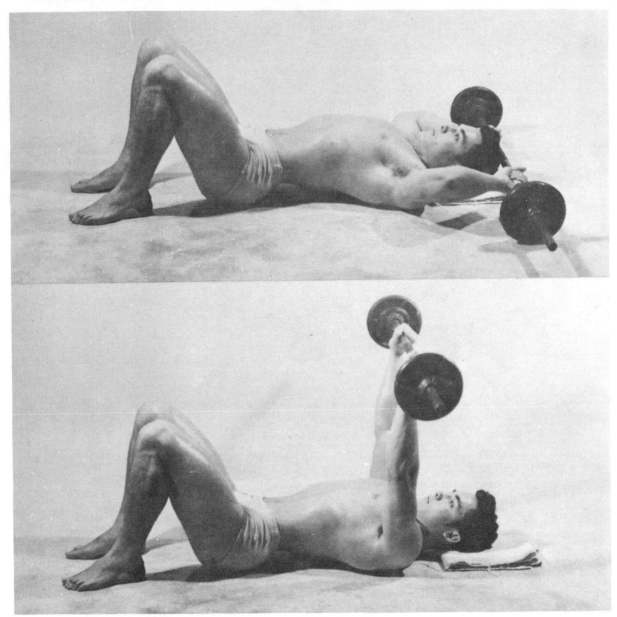

Fig. 160 (upper)   Fig. 161 (lower)

Place a small pillow or blanket under your head when you lie down. Lie flat on your back, with the bar behind your head. Begin this exercise *with the bar only*. Later, you will add weights, as shown in these photographs. Raise your knees and press the calves against the back of your thighs (the soles of your feet should be flat on the floor). Grasp the weight behind your head, shoulder width apart, pull it toward you (*Fig. 160*), and press

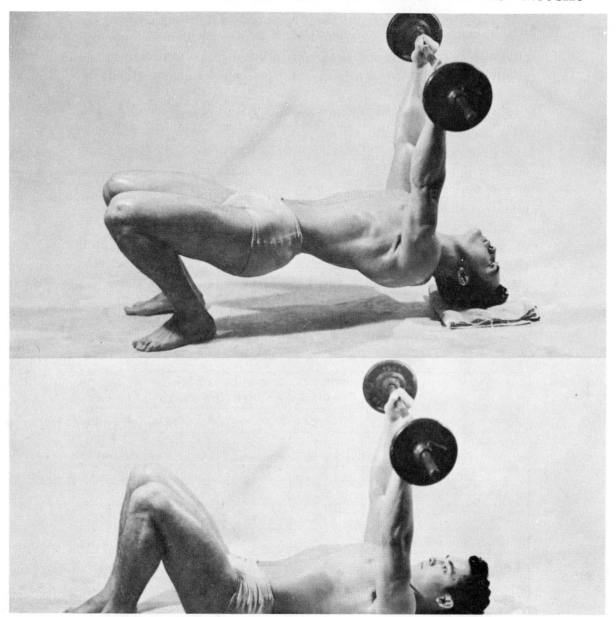

Fig. 162 (upper)   Fig. 163 (lower)

it overhead (*Fig. 161*). Then, bring your head back and arch your body, until it forms a bridge (*Fig. 162*). Now, lower your body to the floor, keeping the weight overhead (*Fig. 163*). Repeat 10 times. After several weeks, add one movement each week until you reach a total of 15. For further development, add a total of 5 pounds, and begin again with 10 repetitions.

Here's power for you

These charts help you keep a record of muscular development. Before you begin training, fill in your measurements on *Chart A* in the column, "Before Training." Take your measurements after 3 months, 6 months, and one year, and note them in the appropriate columns.

Chart B (page 127) is your progress record of all exercises. Before you begin an exercise, note the date, the number of repetitions, and weights (if any) in the first 3 columns. This chart will help you keep a systematic record of your progress. Use it and do not rely on your memory. When the charts are filled up, make your own, following the same form in the book.

Page 128 provides space for photographs you might wish to take before and after the complete training program. The best size photographs are 5″ x 7″ or 4″ x 5″ prints. You might also take a smaller photo, and have it enlarged to the size you want. To mount these prints in the book, use rubber cement. A small jar can be purchased at any stationery store or artist supply shop.

CHART A

	BEFORE TRAINING		AT END OF 3 MONTHS		AT END OF 6 MONTHS		AT END OF 1 YEAR	
	DATE	MEAS.	DATE	MEAS.	DATE	MEAS.	DATE	MEAS.
Height								
Weight								
Neck								
Chest								
Right arm – upper								
Left arm – upper								
Right forearm								
Left forearm								
Right wrist								
Waist								
Hips								
Right thigh								
Right calf								
Right ankle								

CHART B – YOUR PROGRESS RECORD FOR EACH EXERCISE

	Page	Date	Wt.	Rept.	Date	Wt.	Rept.	Date	Wt.	Rept.	Date	Wt.	Rept.	Date	Wt.	Rept.
CALISTHENICS																
Lower back exercise	38															
Adv. lower back exercise	39															
Resistive neck exercise	40															
Resistive neck exercise	41															
Sit-ups	42															
Leg raise	43															
Knee-bend	44															
Advanced knee-bend	45															
Rise-on-toes	46															
Chinning	48															
Side exercises	49															
Hip exercise	50															
Dipping exercise	52															
Advanced dipping	53															
Bicep exercise	54															
DUMBELL EXERCISES																
2-arm alternate press	56															
2-arm alternate curl	59															
Sit-ups (advanced)	60															
Leg-raise	61															
Knee-bend	64															
Pull-over	65															
Dead weight lift	66															
Shoulder shrug	69															
2-arm alternate bench press	70															
Lateral bench press	71															
One-arm rowing motion	72															
One-arm press	74															
Front lateral raise	76															
Side exercise	77															
Bend-over lateral raise	78															
Side lateral raise	79															
One-arm curl	80															
Bend-over one-arm curl	81															
Wrestler's bridge	82															
PULLEY EXERCISES																
Latissimus dorsi exercise	86															
2-arm press	87															
One-arm curl	88															
One-arm curl variation	89															
Back neck muscles	90															
Front neck muscles	91															
One-arm front lateral raise	93															
One-arm side lateral raise	94															
Back deltoid exercise	95															
Tricep exercise	96															
Pectoral muscles exercise	97															

CHART B – YOUR PROGRESS RECORD FOR EACH EXERCISE

	Page	Date	Wt.	Rept.	Date	Wt.	Rept.	Date	Wt.	Rept.	Date	Wt.	Rept.	Date	Wt.	Rept.
BARBELL EXERCISES																
2-arm press	102															
2-arm curl	104															
Sit-ups	106															
Leg-raise	107															
Knee-bend	108															
2-arm pull-over	110															
Bench press	111															
Side exercise	113															
Dead lift	114															
Shoulder shrug	116															
Upright rowing	118															
2-arm press behind neck	119															
Rise-on-toes	120															
2-arm rowing motion	121															
Front lateral raise	122															
Wrestler's bridge	124															